ADVANCED PAEDIATRIC LIFE SUPPORT

ADVANCED PAEDIATRIC LIFE SUPPORT

The Practical Approach

Advanced Life Support Group

BMJ

Published by the BMJ Publishing Group
Tavistock Square, London WC1H 9JR

First published 1993

British Library Cataloguing in Publication Data
A catalogue record for this book is available from the British Library

ISBN 0-7279-0792-1

Typeset, printed and bound in Great Britain by
Latimer Trend & Company Ltd, Plymouth

PREFACE

Advanced Paediatric Life Support: The Practical Approach was written to improve the emergency care of children, and has been developed by a number of paediatricians, paediatric surgeons, accident and emergency specialists, and anaesthetists from several UK centres. It is the core text for the ALPS (UK) course, and will also be of value to medical and allied personnel unable to attend the course. It is designed to include all the common emergencies, and also covers a number of less common diagnoses that are amenable to good initial treatment. The remit is the first hour of care, because it is during this time that the subsequent course of the child is set.

The book is divided into six parts. Part I introduces the subject by discussing the causes of childhood emergencies, the reasons why children need to be treated differently, and the ways in which a seriously ill child can be recognised quickly. Part II deals with the techniques of life support. Both basic and advanced techniques are covered, and there is a separate section on neonatal resuscitation. Part III deals with children who present with serious illness. Shock is dealt with in detail, because recognition and treatment can be particularly difficult. Cardiac and respiratory emergencies, and coma and convulsions, are also discussed. Part IV concentrates on the child who has been seriously injured. Injury is the most common cause of death in the 1–14 year age group and the importance of this topic cannot be overemphasised. Part V gives practical guidance on performing the procedures mentioned elsewhere in the text. Finally, Part VI (the appendices) deals with other areas of importance.

Emergencies in children generate a great deal of anxiety – in the child, the parents, and in the medical and nursing staff who have to deal with them. We hope that this book will shed some light on the subject of paediatric emergency care, and that it will raise the standard of paediatric life support. An understanding of the contents will allow doctors, nurses, and paramedics dealing with seriously ill and injured children to approach their care with confidence.

Kevin Mackway-Jones
Elizabeth Molyneux
Barbara Phillips
Susan Wieteska
(*Editorial Board*)

January 1993

ACKNOWLEDGEMENTS

A great many people have put a lot of work into the production of this book, and the accompanying advanced life support course. The editors would like to thank all the contributors for their efforts.

We are greatly indebted to Helen Carruthers and Mary Harrison MMAA for producing the excellent line drawings that illustrate the text.

Finally, we would like to thank, in advance, those of you who will attend the Advanced Paediatric Life Support (UK) course; no doubt, you will have much constructive criticism to offer.

CONTENTS

CONTENTS

PART V: PRACTICAL PROCEDURES

PART VI: APPENDICES

WORKING GROUP

J. Fothergill	Accident and Emergency Medicine, London
K. Mackway-Jones	Accident and Emergency Medicine, Manchester
E. Molyneux	Paediatric Accident and Emergency, Liverpool
P. Oakley	Anaesthesia/Trauma, Stoke on Trent
B. Phillips	Paediatric Accident and Emergency, Manchester
J. Walker	Paediatric Surgery, Sheffield
S. Wieteska	Course Co-ordinator, Manchester

CONTRIBUTORS

R. Appleton	Paediatric Neurology, Liverpool
I. Barker	Paediatric Anaesthesia, Sheffield
D. Bickerstaff	Paediatric Orthopaedics, Sheffield
R. Bingham	Paediatric Anaesthesia, London
P. Brennan	Paediatric Accident and Emergency Medicine, Sheffield
H. Carty	Paediatric Radiology, Liverpool
M. Clarke	Paediatric Neurology, Manchester
J. Couriel	Paediatric Respiratory Medicine, Manchester
J. Fothergill	Accident and Emergency Medicine, London
E. Ladusans	Paediatric Cardiology, Manchester
S. Levene	Child Accident Prevention Trust, London
M. Lewis	Paediatric Nephrology, Manchester
J. Leggate	Paediatric Neurosurgery, Manchester
K. Mackway-Jones	Accident and Emergency Medicine, Manchester
E. Molyneux	Paediatric Accident and Emergency Medicine, Liverpool
A. Nunn	Pharmacy, Liverpool
P. Oakley	Anaesthesia/Trauma, Stoke on Trent
B. Phillips	Paediatric Accident and Emergency, Manchester

CONTRIBUTORS

J. Robson   Paediatric Accident and Emergency Medicine, Liverpool

D. Sims   Neonatology, Manchester

A. Sprigg   Paediatric Radiology, Sheffield

J. Walker   Paediatric Surgery, Sheffield

S. Wieteska   Course Co-ordinator, Manchester

M. Williams   Accident and Emergency Medicine, York

B. Wilson   Paediatric Radiology, Manchester

PART

I

INTRODUCTION

1

Introduction

CAUSES OF DEATH IN CHILDHOOD

As can be seen from Table 1.1, the greatest mortality during childhood occurs in the first year of life with the highest death rate of all happening in the first month.

Table 1.1. Number of deaths by age group

Age group	Number of deaths
0–28 days	3027
4–52 weeks	2078
1–4 years	955
5–14 years	1128

England and Wales, 1991, Office of Population Censuses and Surveys (OPCS).

The causes of death vary with age as shown in Table 1.2. In the newborn period the most common causes are congenital abnormalities and factors associated with prematurity, such as respiratory immaturity, cerebral haemorrhage, and infection due to immaturity of the immune response.

From 1 month to 1 year of age the condition known as "cot death" is the most common cause of death. Some victims of this condition have previously unrecognised respiratory or metabolic disease, but some have no specific cause of death found at detailed postmortem examination. This latter group is described as suffering from the sudden infant death syndrome. The next most common causes in this age group are congenital abnormalities and infections (Table 1.2).

Table 1.2. Common causes of death by age group

Cause	Number of deaths* at 4–52 weeks	1–4 years	5–14 years
Cot death	880 (42)	0 (0)	0 (0)
Congenital abnormality	349 (18)	194 (20)	116 (10)
Infection	279 (13)	143 (15)	59 (5)
Trauma	86 (4)	211 (22)	382 (34)
Neoplasms	16 (1)	118 (12)	237 (21)

England and Wales, 1991, OPCS.
* Numbers in parentheses are the percentage.

3

INTRODUCTION

After 1 year of age trauma is the most frequent cause of death, and remains so until well into adult life. Deaths from trauma have been described as falling into three groups. In the first group there is overwhelming damage at the time of trauma, and the injury caused is incompatible with life; children with such massive injuries will die within minutes whatever is done. Those in the second group die because of progressive respiratory failure, circulatory insufficiency, or raised intracranial pressure secondary to the effects of injury; death occurs within a few hours if no treatment is administered, but may be avoided if treatment is prompt and effective. The final group consists of late deaths due to infection or multiple organ failure. The trimodal distribution of trauma deaths is illustrated in Figure 1.1.

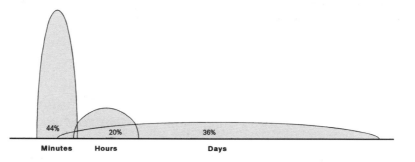

Figure 1.1. Trimodal distribution of deaths from trauma

Only a minority of childhood deaths, such as those due to unresponsive end-stage neoplastic disease, are expected and "managed". Even children with potentially fatal diseases such as complex congenital heart disease, inborn errors of metabolism, or cystic fibrosis have an expectation of "cure" by transplant or gene therapy. The approach to these children is to treat vigorously incidental illnesses (such as respiratory infections) to which many are especially prone. Therefore, some children presenting to hospital with serious life-threatening illness also have an underlying chronic disease.

PATHWAYS LEADING TO CARDIORESPIRATORY ARREST

Cardiac arrest in infancy and childhood is rarely due to primary cardiac disease. This is different from the adult situation where the primary arrest is often cardiac, and cardiorespiratory function may remain near normal until the moment of arrest. In childhood most cardiac arrests are secondary to hypoxia, underlying causes including birth asphyxia, epiglottitis, inhalation of foreign body, bronchiolitis, asthma, and pneumothorax. Respiratory arrest also occurs secondary to neurological dysfunction such as that caused by some poisons or during convulsions. Raised intracranial pressure (ICP) due to head injury or acute encephalopathy eventually leads to respiratory arrest, but severe neuronal damage has already been sustained before the arrest occurs.

Whatever the cause, by the time of cardiac arrest the child has had a period of respiratory insufficiency which will have caused hypoxia and respiratory acidosis. The combination of hypoxia and acidosis causes cell damage and death (particularly in more sensitive organs such as the brain, liver, and kidney), before myocardial damage is severe enough to cause cardiac arrest.

Most other cardiac arrests are secondary to circulatory failure (shock). This will have resulted either from fluid or blood loss, or from fluid maldistribution within the circulatory system. The former may be due to gastroenteritis, burns, or trauma whilst the latter is often caused by sepsis, heart failure, or anaphylaxis. As all organs are

4

deprived of essential nutrients and oxygen as shock progresses to cardiac arrest, circulatory failure, like respiratory failure, causes tissue hypoxia and acidosis. In fact, both pathways may occur in the same condition. The pathways leading to cardiac arrest in children are summarised in Figure 1.2.

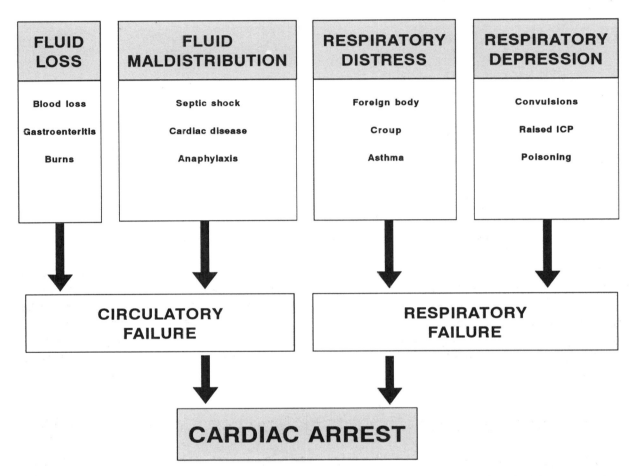

Figure 1.2. Pathways leading to cardiac arrest in childhood (with examples of underlying causes)

The worst outcome is in children who have had an out-of-hospital arrest and who arrive apnoeic and pulseless. These children have a poor chance of intact neurological survival. There has often been a prolonged period of hypoxia and ischaemia before the start of adequate cardiopulmonary resuscitation. Earlier recognition of seriously ill children and paediatric cardiopulmonary resuscitation training for the public could improve the outcome for these children.

2

Why treat children differently?

INTRODUCTION

Children are not little adults. The spectrum of diseases that they suffer from is different, and their responses to disease and injury may differ both physically and psychologically. This chapter deals with some specific points that have particular relevance to emergency care.

SIZE

The most obvious reason for treating children differently is their size, and its variation with age.

Weight

The most rapid changes in size occur in the first year of life. An average birth weight of 3·5 kg has increased to 10·3 kg by the age of 1 year. After that time weight increases more slowly until the pubertal growth spurt. This is illustrated in the weight chart for boys shown in Figure 2.1.

As most therapies are given as the dose per kilogram, it is important to get some idea of a child's weight as soon as possible. In the emergency situation this is especially difficult because it is often impracticable to weigh the child. To overcome this problem a number of methods can be used to derive a weight estimate. If the age is known the formula:

$$\text{Weight (kg)} = 2\,(\text{Age} + 4)$$

can be used if the child is aged between 1 and 10 years old. In addition various charts (such as the Oakley chart) are available which allow an approximation of weight to be derived from the age. Finally, the Broselow tape (which relates weight to height) can be used. Whatever the method, it is essential that the carer is sufficiently familiar with it to be able to use it quickly and accurately.

7

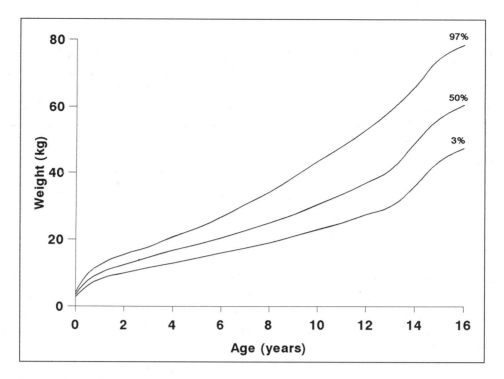

Figure 2.1. Centile chart for weight in boys

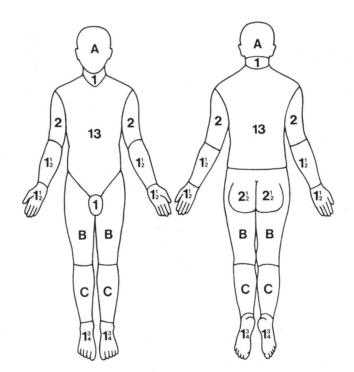

Area indicated	Surface area at				
	0	1 year	5 years	10 years	15 years
A	9·5	8·5	6·5	5·5	4·5
B	2·75	3·25	4·0	4·5	4·5
C	2·5	2·5	2·75	3·0	3·25

Figure 2.2. Body surface area. (Reproduced courtesy of Smith & Nephew Pharmaceuticals Ltd)

Body proportions

The body proportions change with age. This is most graphically illustrated by considering the body surface area (BSA). At birth the head accounts for 19% of BSA; this falls to 9% by the age of 15 years. Figure 2.2 shows these changes.

The BSA to weight ratio decreases with age. Small children, with a high ratio, lose heat more rapidly and consequently are relatively more prone to hypothermia.

Certain specific changes in body proportions also have a bearing on emergency care. For example, the relatively large head and short neck of the infant tend to cause neck flexion and this, together with the relatively large tongue, make airway care difficult. Specific problems such as this are highlighted in the relevant chapters.

ANATOMY AND PHYSIOLOGY

In addition to the general considerations of size, particular anatomical and physiological features, and the way they change with increasing age, can have a bearing on emergency care. Although there are changes in most areas, the most important from this perspective are those that occur in the respiratory and cardiovascular systems. These are discussed in more detail below.

Anatomy

Airway

Anatomical features outside the airway have some relevance to its care. As mentioned above the head is large and the neck short, tending to cause neck flexion. The face and mandible are small and teeth or orthodontic appliances may be loose. The relatively large tongue not only tends to obstruct the airway in an unconscious child, but may also impede the view at laryngoscopy. Finally, the floor of the mouth is easily compressible, requiring care in the positioning of fingers when holding the jaw for airway positioning. These features are summarised in Figure 2.3.

The anatomy of the airway itself changes with age, and consequently different problems affect different age groups. Infants less than 6 months old are obligate nasal breathers. As the narrow nasal passages are easily obstructed by mucus secretions, and upper respiratory tract infections are common in this age group, these children are at particular risk of airway compromise. In 3 to 8 year olds adenotonsillar hypertrophy is a problem. This not only tends to cause obstruction, but also causes difficulty when the nasal route is used to pass pharyngeal, gastric, or tracheal tubes.

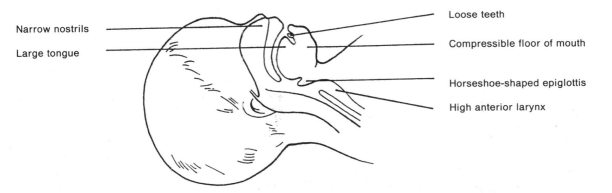

Narrow nostrils

Large tongue

Loose teeth

Compressible floor of mouth

Horseshoe-shaped epiglottis

High anterior larynx

Figure 2.3. Summary of significant upper airway anatomy

In all young children the epiglottis is horseshoe-shaped, and projects posteriorly at 45° making tracheal intubation more difficult. This, together with the fact that the larynx is high and anterior (at the level of the second and third cervical vertebrae in the infant, compared with the fifth and sixth vertebrae in the adult), means that it is easier to intubate an infant using a straight-blade laryngoscope. The cricoid ring is the narrowest part of the upper airway (as opposed to the larynx in an adult). The narrow cross-sectional area at this point, together with the fact that the cricoid ring is lined by pseudostratified ciliated epithelium loosely bound to areolar tissue, makes it particularly susceptible to oedema. As endotracheal tube cuffs tend to lie at this level, uncuffed tubes are preferred in pre-pubertal children.

The trachea is short and soft. Over-extension of the neck may therefore cause tracheal compression. The short trachea and the symmetry of the carinal angles mean that, not only is tube displacement more likely, but also a tube or a foreign body is just as likely to be displaced into the left as the right main-stem bronchus.

Breathing

The lungs are relatively immature at birth. The air–tissue interface has a relatively small total surface area in the infant (less than $3\,m^2$). In addition, there is a tenfold increase in the number of small airways from birth to adulthood.

Both the upper and lower airways are relatively small, and are consequently more easily obstructed. As resistance to flow is inversely proportional to the fourth power of the airway radius (halving the radius increases the resistance sixteenfold), seemingly small obstructions can have significant effects on air entry in children.

Infants rely mainly on diaphragmatic breathing. Their muscles are more likely to fatigue, as they have fewer type I (slow twitch, highly oxidative, fatigue-resistant) fibres compared with adults. Pre-term infants' muscles have even less type I fibres. These children are consequently more prone to respiratory failure.

The ribs lie more horizontally in infants, and therefore contribute less to chest expansion. In the injured child, the compliant chest wall may allow serious parenchymal injuries to occur without necessarily incurring rib fractures. For multiple rib fractures to occur the force must be very large; the parenchymal injury that results is consequently very severe and flail chest is tolerated badly.

Circulation

At birth the two cardiac ventricles are of similar weight; by 2 months of age the RV/LV weight ratio is 0·5. These changes are reflected in the infant's ECG. During the first months of life the right ventricle (RV) dominance is apparent, but by 4–6 months of age the left ventricle (LV) is dominant. As the heart develops during childhood, the sizes of the P wave and QRS complex increase, and the P–R interval and QRS duration become longer.

The child's circulating blood volume is higher per kilogram body weight (70–80 ml/kg) than that of an adult, but the actual volume is small. This means that in infants and small children relatively small absolute amounts of blood loss can be critically important.

Physiology

Airway and breathing

The infant has a relatively greater metabolic rate and oxygen consumption. This is one reason for an increased respiratory rate. However, the tidal volume remains relatively constant in relation to body weight (5–7 ml/kg) through to adulthood. The work of breathing is also relatively unchanged at about 1% of the metabolic rate, although it is increased in the pre-term infant.

10

Table 2.1. Respiratory rate by age

Age (years)	Respiratory rate (breaths per minute)
<1	30–40
2–5	20–30
5–12	15–20
>12	12–16

In the adult, the lung and chest wall contribute equally to the total compliance. In the newborn, most of the impedance to expansion is due to the lung, and is critically dependent on surfactant. The lung compliance increases over the first week of life as fluid is removed from the lung. The child's compliant chest wall leads to prominent sternal recession and rib space indrawing when the airway is obstructed or lung compliance decreases. It also allows the intrathoracic pressure to be less "negative". This reduces small airway patency. As a result, the lung volume is similar to the closing volume (the volume at which small airway closure starts to take place).

At birth, the oxygen dissociation curve is shifted to the left and P_{50} (Po_2 at 50% oxygen saturation) is greatly reduced. This is due to the fact that 70% of the haemoglobin is in the form of HbF; this gradually declines to negligible amounts by the age of 6 months.

Circulation

The infant has a relatively small stroke volume (1·5 ml/kg at birth) but has the highest cardiac index seen at any stage of life (300 ml/kg). Cardiac index decreases with age and is 100 ml/kg in adolescence and 70–80 ml/kg in the adult. At the same time the stroke volume increases as the heart gets bigger. As cardiac output is the product of stroke volume and heart rate, these changes underlie the heart rate changes seen during childhood (shown in Table 2.2).

Table 2.2. Heart rate by age

Age (years)	Heart rate (beats per minute)
<1	110–160
2–5	95–140
5–12	80–120
>12	60–100

As the stroke volume is small and relatively fixed in infants, cardiac output is directly related to heart rate. The practical importance of this is that the response to volume therapy is blunted because stroke volume cannot increase greatly to improve cardiac output. By the age of 2 years myocardial function and response to fluid are similar to those of an adult.

Systemic vascular resistance rises after birth and continues to do so until adulthood is reached. This is reflected in the changes seen in blood pressure – shown in Table 2.3.

Table 2.3. Systolic blood pressure by age

Age (years)	Systolic blood pressure (mmHg)
<1	70–90
2–5	80–100
5–12	90–110
>12	100–120

PSYCHOLOGY

Children who are ill or injured present particular problems during emergency management because of difficulties in communicating with them, and because of the fear that they feel.

Communication

Infants and young children either have no language ability or are still developing their speech. This causes difficulty when symptoms such as pain need to be described. Even children who are usually fluent may remain silent. Information has to be gleaned from the limited verbal communication, and from the many non-verbal cues (such as facial expression and posture) that are available.

Fear

All emergency situations, and many other situations that adults would not classify as emergencies, engender fear in children. This causes additional distress to the child and adds to parental anxiety. Physiological parameters, such as pulse rate and respiratory rate, are altered because of it, and this in turn makes clinical assessment more difficult.

Fear is a particular problem in the pre-school child who often has a "magical" concept of illness and injury. This means that the child may think that the problem has been caused by some bad wish or thought that he or she has had. School-age children and adolescents may have fearsome concepts of what might happen to them because of ideas they have picked up from adult conversation, films, and television.

Knowledge allays fear and it is therefore important to explain things as clearly as possible to the child. Explanations must be phrased in a way that the child can understand. Play can be used to do this (e.g. applying a bandage to a teddy first), and also helps to maintain some semblance of normality in a strange and stressful situation. Finally, parents must be allowed to stay with the child at all times; their absence from the bedside will only add additional fears both to the child and to the parents themselves.

Parents

Summary

- Absolute size and relative body proportions change with age
- Observations on children must be related to their age
- Therapy in children must be related to their age and weight
- The special psychological needs of children must be considered

---

3

Recognition of the seriously ill child

As described in Chapter 1, the outcome for children following cardiac arrest is, in general, very poor. Earlier recognition and management of potential respiratory, circulatory, or central neurological failure will reduce mortality and secondary morbidity. This chapter describes the physical signs that should be used for rapid assessment of children.

RECOGNITION OF POTENTIAL RESPIRATORY FAILURE

Work of breathing

The degree of increase in the work of breathing allows clinical assessment of the severity of respiratory disease. It is important to assess the following.

Respiratory rate

At rest tachypnoea indicates that increased ventilation is needed because of either lung or airway disease, or metabolic acidosis. Normal respiratory rates at differing ages are shown in Table 3.1.

Table 3.1. Respiratory rate by age

Age (years)	Respiratory rate (breaths per minute)
<1	30–40
2–5	20–30
5–12	15–20
>12	12–16

Recession

Intercostal, subcostal, or sternal recession shows increased work of breathing. This sign is more easily seen in younger infants as they have a more compliant chest wall. Its presence in older children (i.e. over 6 or 7 years) suggests severe respiratory problems. The degree of recession gives an indication of the severity of respiratory difficulty.

13

Inspiratory or expiratory noises

An inspiratory noise while breathing (stridor) is a sign of laryngeal or tracheal obstruction. In severe obstruction the stridor may also occur in expiration, but the inspiratory component is usually more pronounced. Wheezing indicates lower airway narrowing and is more pronounced in expiration. A prolonged expiratory phase also indicates lower airway narrowing. The volume of the noise is not an indicator of severity.

Grunting

Grunting is produced by exhalation against a partially closed glottis. It is an attempt to generate a positive end-expiratory pressure and prevent airway collapse at the end of expiration in children with "stiff" lungs. This is a sign of severe respiratory distress and is characteristically seen in infants.

Accessory muscle use

As in adult life, the sternomastoid muscle may be used as an accessory respiratory muscle when the work of breathing is increased. In infants this may cause the head to bob up and down with each breath, making it ineffectual.

Flare of the alae nasi

Flaring of the alae nasi is seen in infants with respiratory distress.

Exceptions

There may be absent or decreased evidence of increased work of breathing in three circumstances:
1. In the infant or child who has had severe respiratory problems for some time, fatigue may occur and the signs of increased work of breathing will decrease. *Exhaustion is a pre-terminal sign.*
2. Children with cerebral depression from raised intracranial pressure, poisoning or encephalopathy will have respiratory inadequacy without increased work of breathing. The respiratory inadequacy in this case is caused by decreased respiratory drive.
3. Children who have neuromuscular disease (such as Werdnig–Hoffman disease or muscular dystrophy) may present in respiratory failure without increased work of breathing.

The diagnosis of respiratory failure in such children is made by observing the effectiveness of breathing, and looking for other signs of respiratory inadequacy. These are discussed in the text.

Effectiveness of breathing

Auscultation of the chest will give an indication of the amount of air being inspired and expired. *A silent chest is an extremely worrying sign.* Similarly, observations of the degree of *chest expansion* (or, in infants, abdominal excursion) adds useful information.

Pulse oximetry can be used to measure the arterial oxygen saturation (Sao_2). The instruments are less accurate when Sao_2 is less than 70%, when shock is present, and in the presence of carboxyhaemoglobin.

Effects of respiratory inadequacy on other organs

Heart rate

Hypoxia produces tachycardia in the older infant and child. Anxiety and a fever will also contribute to tachycardia. Severe or prolonged hypoxia leads to bradycardia. *This is a pre-terminal sign.*

Skin colour

Hypoxia (via catecholamine release) produces vasoconstriction and skin pallor. *Cyanosis is a late and pre-terminal sign of hypoxia.* By the time central cyanosis is visible in acute respiratory disease, the patient is close to respiratory arrest. In the anaemic child cyanosis may never be visible despite profound hypoxia.

Mental status

The hypoxic or hypercapnic child will be agitated and/or drowsy. Gradually drowsiness increases and eventually consciousness is lost. These extremely useful and important signs are often more difficult to detect in small infants. The parents may say that the infant is just "not himself". The doctor must assess the child's state of alertness by gaining eye contact, and noting the response to voice and, if necessary, to painful stimuli. A generalised muscular hypotonia also accompanies hypoxic cerebral depression.

RECOGNITION OF POTENTIAL CIRCULATORY FAILURE (SHOCK)

Cardiovascular status

Heart rate

The heart rate initially increases in shock due to catecholamine release and as compensation for decreased stroke volume. The rate, particularly in small infants, may be extremely high (up to 220 per minute). Normal rates are shown in Table 3.2.

Table 3.2. Heart rate by age

Age (years)	Heart rate (beats per minute)
<1	110–160
2–5	95–140
5–12	80–120
>12	60–100

Pulse volume

Although blood pressure is maintained until shock is very severe, an indication of perfusion can be gained by palpation of both peripheral and central pulses. Absent peripheral pulses and weak central pulses are serious signs of advanced shock, and indicate that hypotension is already present.

Capillary refill

Following cutaneous pressure on a digit for 5 seconds, capillary refill should occur within 2 seconds. A slower refill time than this indicates poor skin perfusion.

Blood pressure

Hypotension is a late and pre-terminal sign of circulatory failure. Once a child's blood pressure has fallen cardiac arrest is imminent. Expected systolic blood pressure can be estimated by the formula:

$$\text{Blood pressure} = 80 + (\text{Age in years} \times 2)$$

15

Normal systolic pressures are shown in Table 3.3.

Table 3.3. Systolic blood pressure by age

Age (years)	Systolic blood pressure (mmHg)
<1	70–90
2–5	80–100
5–12	90–110
>12	100–120

Use of the correct cuff size is crucial if an accurate blood pressure measurement is to be obtained. This caveat applies both to auscultatory and to oscillometric devices.

Effects of circulatory inadequacy on other organs

Respiratory system

A rapid respiration rate with an increased tidal volume, but without recession, is characteristic of acidosis resulting from circulatory failure.

Skin

Mottled, cold, pale skin peripherally indicates poor perfusion. A line of coldness may be perceived to move centrally as circulatory failure progresses.

Mental status

Agitation and then drowsiness leading to unconsciousness are characteristic of circulatory failure. Initial agitation is caused by catecholamine release, whereas subsequent drowsiness is caused by poor cerebral perfusion.

Urinary output

A urine output of less than 1 ml/kg/hour in children and less than 2 ml/kg/hour in infants indicates inadequate renal perfusion during shock. A history of oliguria or anuria should be sought.

RECOGNITION OF POTENTIAL CENTRAL NEUROLOGICAL FAILURE

Neurological assessment should only be performed after airway (A), breathing (B), and circulation (C) have been assessed and treated. There are no neurological problems that take priority over ABC.

Both respiratory and circulatory failure will have central neurological effects. Conversely, some conditions with direct central neurological effects (such as meningitis, raised intracranial pressure from trauma, and status epilepticus) may also have respiratory and circulatory consequences.

Neurological function

Conscious level

A rapid assessment of conscious level can be made by assigning the patient to one of the categories shown in the box.

A	ALERT
V	responds to VOICE
P	responds to PAIN
U	UNRESPONSIVE

The painful stimulus should be delivered either by pinching a digit or by pulling frontal hair. A child who is unconscious or who only responds to pain has a significant degree of coma.

Posture

Many children who are suffering from a serious illness in any system are hypotonic. Stiff posturing such as that shown by decorticate (flexed arms, extended legs) or decerebrate (extended arms, extended legs) children is a sign of serious brain dysfunction.

Pupils

Many drugs and cerebral lesions have effects on pupil size and reactions. However, the most important pupillary signs to seek are dilatation, unreactivity, and inequality, which indicate possible serious brain disorders.

Respiratory effects of central neurological failure

There are several recognisable breathing pattern abnormalities with raised intracranial pressure. However, they are often changeable and may vary from hyperventilation to Cheyne–Stokes breathing to apnoea. The presence of an abnormal respiratory pattern in a patient with coma suggests mid- or hind-brain dysfunction.

Circulatory effects of central neurological failure

Systemic hypertension with sinus bradycardia (Cushing's response) indicates compression of the medulla oblongata caused by herniation of the cerebellar tonsils through the foramen magnum. *This is a late and pre-terminal sign.*

Summary: the rapid assessment of an infant or child

       Airway and Breathing
          Work of breathing
          Respiratory rate/rhythm
          Stridor/wheeze
          Auscultation
          Skin colour
       Circulation
          Heart rate
          Pulse volume
          Capillary refill
          Skin temperature
       Disability
          Mental status/conscious level
          Posture
          Pupils

The whole assessment should take less than a minute

Once airway (A), breathing (B), and circulation (C) are clearly recognised as being stable or have been stabilised, then definitive management of the underlying condition can proceed. During definitive management reassessment of ABCD at frequent intervals will be necessary to assess progress and detect deterioration.

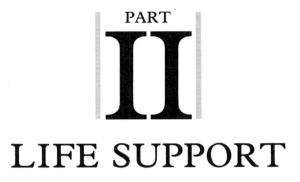

LIFE SUPPORT

4

Basic life support

Paediatric basic life support (BLS) is not simply a scaled-down version of that provided for adults. Although the general principles are the same, specific techniques are required if the optimum support is to be given. The exact techniques employed need to be varied according to the size of the child. A somewhat artificial line is generally drawn between infants (less than 1 year old) and small children (less than 8 years old), and this chapter follows that approach.

By applying the basic techniques described, a single rescuer can support the vital respiratory and circulatory functions of a collapsed child with no equipment.

Basic life support is the foundation on which advanced life support is built. Therefore it is essential that all advanced life support providers are proficient at basic techniques, and that they are capable of ensuring that basic support is provided continuously and well during resuscitation.

ASSESSMENT AND TREATMENT

Once the child has been approached correctly and a simple test for unresponsiveness has been carried out, assessment and treatment follow the familiar A, B, C pattern. The overall sequence of basic life support in paediatric cardiopulmonary arrest is summarised in Figure 4.1.

The SAFE approach

Additional help should be summoned rapidly. Furthermore, it is essential that the rescuer does not become a second victim, and that the child is removed from continuing danger as quickly as possible. These considerations should precede the initial airway assessment. They are summarised in Figure 4.2.

Are you alright?

The initial simple assessment of responsiveness consists of asking the child "Are you alright?", and *gently* shaking him or her by the shoulders. Infants and very small

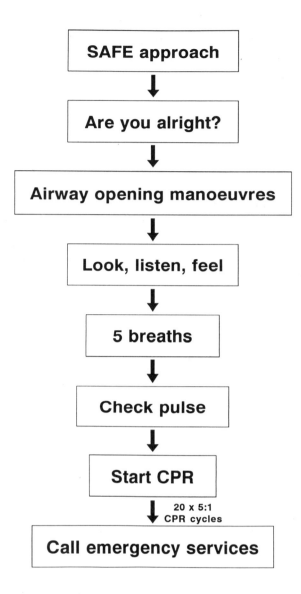

Figure 4.1. The overall sequence of basic life support in cardiopulmonary arrest. (CPR=cardiopulmonary resuscitation)

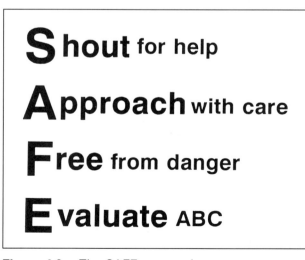

Figure 4.2. The SAFE approach

children who cannot talk yet, and older children who are very scared, are unlikely to reply meaningfully, but may make some sound or open their eyes to the rescuer's voice.

In cases associated with trauma, the neck and spine should be immobilised during this manoeuvre. This is achieved by placing one hand firmly on the forehead, while one of the child's arms is shaken gently.

Airway (A)

An obstructed airway may be the primary problem, and correction of the obstruction can result in recovery without further intervention.

If a child is having difficulty breathing, but is conscious, then transport to hospital should be arranged as quickly as possible. A child will often find the best position to maintain his or her own airway, and should not be forced to adopt a position that may be less comfortable. Attempts to improve a partially maintained airway in an environment where immediate advanced support is not available can be dangerous, because total obstruction may occur.

If the child is not breathing it may be because the airway has been blocked by the tongue falling back to obstruct the pharynx. An attempt to open the airway should be made using the head tilt/chin lift manoeuvre. The rescuer places the hand nearest to the child's head on the forehead, and applies pressure to tilt the head back gently. The desirable degrees of tilt are: *neutral* in the infant and *sniffing* in the child.

These are shown in Figures 4.3 and 4.4.

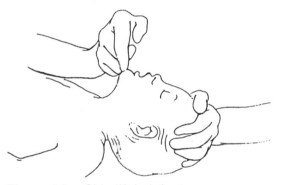

Figure 4.3. Chin lift in infants

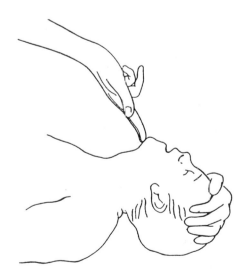

Figure 4.4. Chin lift in children

The fingers of the other hand should then be placed under the chin and the chin should be lifted upwards. Care should be taken not to injure the soft tissue by gripping too hard. As this action can close the child's mouth, it may be necessary to use the thumb of the same hand to part the lips slightly.

The patency of the airway should then be assessed. This is done by:

LOOKing   for chest movement
LISTENing   for breath sounds
FEELing   for breath

and is best achieved by the rescuer placing his or her face above the child's, with the ear over the nose, the cheek over the mouth, and the eyes looking along the line of the chest.

If the head tilt/chin lift has been unsuccessful or is contraindicated, then the jaw thrust manoeuvre can be performed. This is achieved by placing two or three fingers under the angle of the mandible bilaterally, and lifting the jaw upwards. This technique may be easier if the rescuer's elbows are resting on the same surface as the child is lying on. A small degree of head tilt may also be applied. This is shown in Figure 4.5.

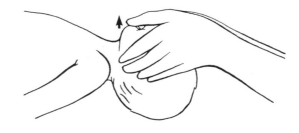

Figure 4.5.   Jaw thrust

As before the success or failure of the intervention is assessed using the

LOOK
LISTEN
FEEL

technique described above.

It should be noted that, if there is a history of trauma, then the head tilt/chin lift manoeuvre may exacerbate cervical spine injury. The safest airway intervention in these circumstances is jaw thrust without head tilt. Proper cervical spine control can only be achieved in such cases by a second rescuer maintaining in-line cervical stabilisation throughout.

The finger sweep technique often recommended in adults should not be used in children. The child's soft palate is easily damaged and bleeding from within the mouth can worsen the situation. Furthermore, foreign bodies may be forced further down the airway; they can become lodged below the vocal cords (vocal folds) and be even more difficult to remove.

If a foreign body is not obvious, inspection should be done under direct vision in hospital and, if appropriate, removal should be attempted using Magill's forceps.

Breathing (B)

If the airway opening techniques described above do not result in the resumption of breathing, exhaled air resuscitation should be commenced.

Five initial rescue breaths should be given.

While the airway is kept open as described above, the rescuer breathes in and seals his or her mouth around the victim's mouth, or mouth and nose as shown in Figure 4.6. If the mouth alone is used then the nose should be pinched closed using the thumb and index fingers of the hand that is maintaining head tilt. Slow exhalation (1–1·5 seconds) by the rescuer should result in the victim's chest rising.

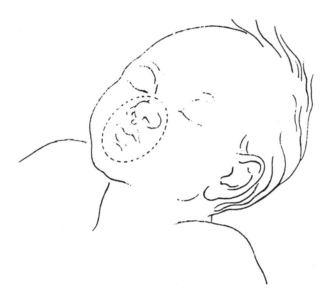

Figure 4.6. Mouth-to-mouth-and-nose in a small child

As children vary in size only general guidance can be given regarding the volume and pressure of inflation (see the box).

General guidance for exhaled air resuscitation

- The chest should be seen to rise
- Inflation pressure may be higher because the airway is small
- Slow breaths at the lowest pressure reduce gastric distension

---

If the chest does not rise then the airway is not clear. The usual cause is failure to apply correctly the airway opening techniques discussed above. Thus the first thing to do is to readjust the head tilt/chin lift position, and try again. If this does not work jaw thrust should be tried. It is quite possible for a single rescuer to open the airway using this technique and perform exhaled air resuscitation; however, if two rescuers are present one should maintain the airway whilst the other breathes for the child.

Failure of both head tilt/chin and jaw thrust should lead to the suspicion that a foreign body is causing the obstruction, and the appropriate action should be taken (see below).

Circulation (C)

Once the initial five breaths have been given as above, attention should be turned to the circulation.

Assessment

Inadequacy of the circulation is recognised by the absence of a central pulse for 5 seconds or by the presence of a pulse at an insufficient rate. In children, as in adults, the carotid artery in the neck can be palpated.

In infants the neck is generally short and fat, and the carotid artery may be difficult to identify. Therefore the brachial artery in the medial aspect of the antecubital fossa (Figure 4.7), or the femoral artery in the groin, should be felt.

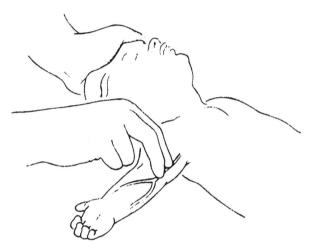

Figure 4.7. Feeling for the brachial pulse

If the pulse is absent for 5 seconds or inadequate (less than 60 beats per minute in infants and small children, and less than 40 beats per minute in larger children), then cardiac compression is required. If the pulse is present and at an adequate rate, but apnoea persists, exhaled air resuscitation must be continued until spontaneous breathing resumes.

The precordial thump is not recommended in children.

Cardiac compression

For the best output the child must be placed lying flat on his or her back, on a hard surface. In infants it is said that the palm of the rescuer's hand can be used for this purpose, but this may prove difficult in practice.

Children vary in size, and the exact nature of the compressions given should reflect this. In general, infants (less than 1 year) require a different technique from small children. In children over 8 years of age, the method used in adults can be applied with appropriate modifications for their size.

Infants As the infant heart is lower with relation to external landmarks when compared to older children and adults, the area of compression is found by imagining a line between the nipples and compressing over the sternum one finger-breadth below this line. Two fingers are used to compress the chest to a depth of approximately 1·5–2·5 cm. This is shown in Figure 4.8. Alternatively, infant cardiac compression can be

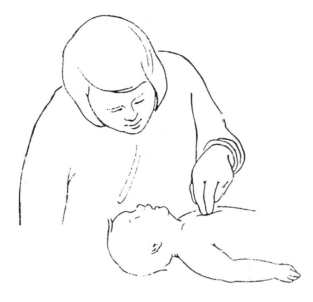

Figure 4.8. Infant chest compression: two-finger technique

achieved using the hand-encircling technique: the infant is held with both the rescuer's hands encircling the chest. The thumbs are placed over the correct part of the sternum (see above) and compression carried out, as shown in Figure 4.9.

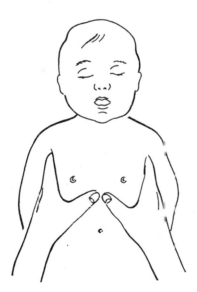

Figure 4.9. Infant chest compression: hand-encircling technique

Small children The area of compression is one finger-breadth above the xiphisternum. The heel of one hand is used to compress the sternum to a depth of approximately 2·5–3·5 cm (Figure 4.10).

27

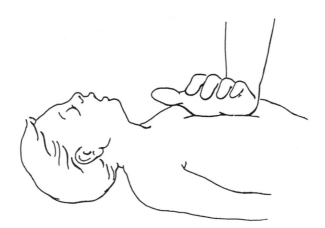

Figure 4.10. Chest compression in small children

Larger children The area of compression is two finger-breadths above the xiphister-num. The heels of both hands are used to compress the sternum to a depth of approximately 3–4·5 cm depending on the size of the child (Figure 4.11).

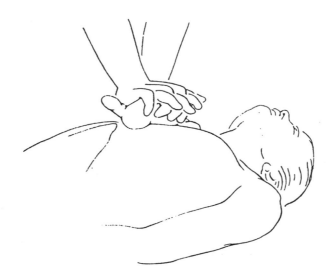

Figure 4.11. Chest compression in older children

Once the correct technique has been chosen and the area for compression identified, five compressions should be given.

Continuing cardiopulmonary resuscitation

A ratio of five compressions to one ventilation is maintained whatever the number of rescuers. As the normal heart rate in infants and children is higher than in adults, the recommended compression rate is also higher at 100 per minute. This equates with a cycle rate of 20 per minute.

If no help has arrived the emergency services must be contacted after 20 full cardiopulmonary resuscitation cycles have been delivered. *Apart from this interruption to summon help, basic life support must not be interrupted unless the child moves or takes a breath.*

28

Any time spent readjusting the airway or re-establishing the correct position for compressions will seriously decrease the number of cycles given per minute. This can be a very real problem for the solo rescuer and there is no easy solution.

The cardiopulmonary resuscitation manoeuvres recommended for infants and children are summarised in Table 4.1.

Table 4.1. Summary of basic life support techniques in infants and children

	Infant	Small child	Larger child
Airway			
Head-tilt position	Neutral	Sniffing	Sniffing
Breathing			
Initial slow breaths	5	5	5
Circulation			
Pulse check	Brachial or femoral	Carotid	Carotid
Landmark	One finger-breadth below nipple line	One finger-breadth above xiphisternum	Two finger-breadths above xiphisternum
Technique	Two fingers or encircling	One hand	Two hands
Depth (cm)	1·5–2·5	2·5–3·5	3–4·5
Cardiopulmonary resuscitation			
Ratio	5:1	5:1	5:1
Cycles per minute	20	20	20

BASIC LIFE SUPPORT AND INFECTION RISK

There have been a few reports of transmission of infectious diseases from casualties to rescuers during mouth-to-mouth resuscitation. The most serious concern in children is meningococcus, and rescuers involved in the resuscitation of the airway in such patients should take standard prophylactic antibiotics (usually rifampicin).

There have been no reported cases of transmission of either hepatitis B or human immunodeficiency virus (HIV) through mouth-to-mouth ventilation. Blood-to-blood contact is the single most important route of transmission of these viruses, and in non-trauma resuscitations the risks are negligible. Sputum, saliva, sweat, tears, urine, and vomit are low-risk fluids. Precautions should be taken, if possible, in cases where there might be contact with blood, semen, vaginal secretions, cerebrospinal fluid, pleural and peritoneal fluids, and amniotic fluid. Precautions are also recommended if any bodily secretion contains visible blood. Devices that prevent direct contact between the rescuer and the victim (such as resuscitation masks) can be used to lower risk; gauze swabs or any other porous material placed over the victim's mouth is of no benefit in this regard.

The number of children in the UK with AIDS or HIV-1 infection in June 1992 was estimated at 501, whereas the number of adults similarly affected was estimated at 23 806 (a ratio of 1:47). If transmission of HIV-1 does occur, it is therefore much more likely to be from adult rescuer to child rather than the other way around.

Although practice manikins have not been shown to be a source of infection, regular cleaning is recommended and should be carried out as shown in the manufacturer's instructions.

THE CHOKING CHILD

Introduction

The vast majority of deaths from foreign body aspiration occur in pre-school children. Virtually anything may be inhaled. The diagnosis is very rarely clear-cut, but should be suspected if the onset of respiratory compromise is sudden and is associated with coughing, gagging, and stridor. Airway obstruction may also occur with infections such as acute epiglottitis and croup. In such cases, attempts to relieve the obstruction using the methods described below are dangerous. Children with known or suspected infectious causes of obstruction, and those who are still breathing and in whom the cause of obstruction is unclear, should be taken to hospital urgently. The treatment of these children is dealt with in Chapter 9.

The physical methods of clearing the airway, described below, should therefore only be performed if:

1. The diagnosis of foreign body aspiration is clear-cut, and dyspnoea is increasing or apnoea has occurred.
2. Head tilt/chin lift and jaw thrust have failed to open the airway of an apnoeic child.

Infants

Abdominal thrusts may cause intra-abdominal injury in infants. Therefore a combination of back blows and chest thrusts is recommended for the relief of foreign body obstruction in this age group.

The baby is placed along one of the rescuer's arms in a head-down position. The rescuer then rests his or her arm along the thigh, and delivers five back blows with the heel of the free hand.

If the obstruction is not relieved the baby is turned over and laid along the rescuer's thigh, still in a head-down position. Five chest thrusts are given – using the same landmarks as for cardiac compression but slower. If an infant is too large to allow the single-arm technique described above to be used, then the same manoeuvres can be performed by lying the baby across the rescuer's lap. These techniques are shown in Figures 4.12 and 4.13.

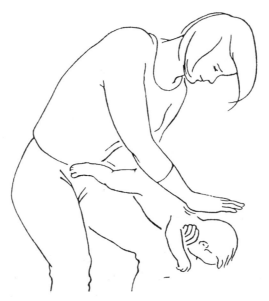

Figure 4.12. Back blows in an infant

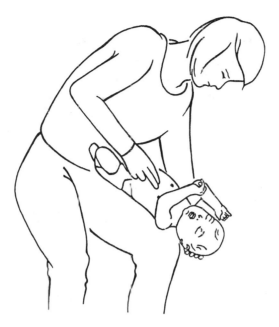

Figure 4.13. Chest thrusts in an infant

Children

Back blows can be used as in infants (Figure 4.14). In the older child the Heimlich manoeuvre can also be used. As in the adult this can be performed with the victim either standing, sitting, kneeling, or lying.

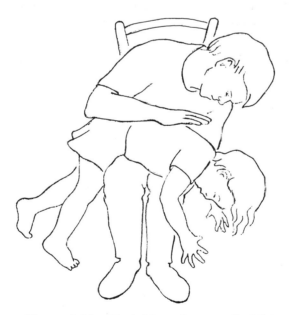

Figure 4.14. Back blows in a small child

If this is to be attempted with the child standing, kneeling, or sitting, the rescuer moves behind the victim and passes his or her arms around the victim's body. Due to the height of children, it may be necessary for an adult to stand the child on a box or other convenient object to carry out the standing manoeuvre effectively. One hand is formed

31

into a fist and placed against the child's abdomen above the umbilicus and below the xiphisternum. The other hand is placed over the fist, and both hands are thrust sharply upwards into the abdomen. This is repeated ten times unless the object causing the obstruction is expelled before then. This technique is shown in Figure 4.15.

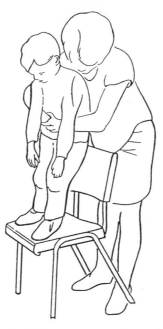

Figure 4.15. Heimlich manoeuvre in a standing child

To carry out the Heimlich manoeuvre in a supine child, the rescuer kneels at his or her feet (Figure 4.16). If the child is large it may be necessary to kneel astride him or her. The heel of one hand is placed against the child's abdomen above the umbilicus and below the xiphisternum. The other hand is placed on top of the first, and both hands are thrust sharply upwards into the abdomen with care being taken to direct the thrust in the midline. This is repeated ten times unless the object causing the obstruction is expelled before then.

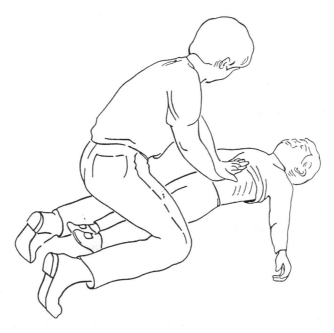

Figure 4.16. Abdominal thrusts

5

Advanced support of the airway and ventilation

Management of airway and breathing has priority in the resuscitation of patients of all ages; the rate at which respiratory function can deteriorate in children is particularly rapid. It is vital that effective resuscitation techniques can be applied quickly and in order of priority. To do so, it is useful to appreciate the differences between adults and children, and essential to be familiar with commonly used equipment. Techniques for obtaining a patent and protected airway, and of achieving adequate ventilation and oxygenation, must be learned and practised. Finally, these techniques must be integrated into a prioritised system of care, planned in advance, to avoid delays and uncertainties in emergency situations.

EQUIPMENT FOR MANAGING THE AIRWAY

The airway equipment indicated in the box should be available in designated resuscitation areas. It is crucial that familiarity with it is gained before it is needed in an emergency situation.

Necessary airway equipment

Suction devices
Pharyngeal airways
Laryngoscopes
Endotracheal tubes, introducers, and connectors
Magill's forceps
Tracheal suction catheters
Cricothyroidotomy cannulae and ventilation systems

Suction devices

In the resuscitation room, the usual suction device is the pipeline vacuum unit. It consists of a suction hose inserted into a wall terminal outlet, a controller (to adjust the vacuum pressure), a reservoir jar, suction tubing, and a suitable sucker nozzle or catheter. In order to aspirate vomit effectively, it should be capable of producing a high negative pressure and a high flow rate, although these can be reduced in non-urgent situations, so as not to cause mucosal injury.

The most useful suction ending is the Yankauer sucker, which is available in both adult and paediatric sizes. The paediatric size has a side hole which can be occluded by a finger, allowing greater control over vacuum pressure. In small infants, a suction catheter and a Y-piece are often preferred, but are less capable of removing vomit.

Portable suction devices are required for resuscitation in remote locations, and for transport to and from the resuscitation room. These are commonly operated by a hand or foot pump.

Pharyngeal airways

There are two main types of pharyngeal airway:

1. Oropharyngeal.
2. Nasopharyngeal.

The oropharyngeal or Guedel airway is used in the obtunded patient to provide a patent airway channel between the tongue and the posterior pharyngeal wall. It may also be used to stabilise the position of an oral endotracheal tube. In the awake patient with an intact gag reflex, it may not be tolerated and may provoke vomiting. It is available in a variety of sizes. A useful rule for estimating size is that the appropriate airway extends from the centre of the mouth to the angle of the jaw when laid on the child's face. An inappropriate size may cause laryngospasm, mucosal trauma or may worsen the airway obstruction. Two techniques for insertion are described in Chapter 21.

The nasopharyngeal airway is often better tolerated than the Guedel airway. It is contraindicated in fractures of the anterior base of the skull. It may also cause significant haemorrhage from the friable, vascular, nasal mucosa. A suitable length can be estimated by measuring from the tip of the nose to the tragus of the ear. An appropriate diameter is one that just fits into the nostril without causing sustained blanching of the alae nasi. As small-sized nasopharyngeal airways are not commercially available, shortened endotracheal tubes may be used.

Laryngoscopes

There are two principal designs of laryngoscope for use in children: the straight-blade and the curved-blade laryngoscope. In general the straight-blade laryngoscope is designed to lift the epiglottis under the tip of the blade, whereas the curved-blade laryngoscope is designed to rest in the vallecula. The straight-blade device can also be placed short of the epiglottis in the vallecula. The advantage of taking the epiglottis is that it cannot then obscure the view of the vocal cords (vocal folds). The advantage of stopping short of the epiglottis is that it causes less stimulation, and is less likely to cause laryngospasm. The blade length should be varied according to the age. It should be noted that it is possible to intubate successfully with a blade that is too long, but not with one that is too short. In general, straight blades are preferred up to the age of 1 year, and many prefer to use them up to the age of 5 years.

It is important to have a spare laryngoscope available, together with spare bulbs and batteries, to overcome equipment failure. In fibreoptic designs, the bulbs are set in the top of the blade handle rather than in the blade itself. This has advantages in terms of bulb protection and the ability to clean the blade after use.

The essential parts of these laryngoscopes are shown in Figures 5.1 and 5.2. The flange is designed to displace the tongue to the left in order to optimise the view of the larynx. Failure to control the tongue adequately in the haste to see the vocal cords may leave a portion of the tongue overhanging the blade. It may still be possible to see the larynx at first, but as soon as the endotracheal tube is placed in the mouth, the view is obscured.

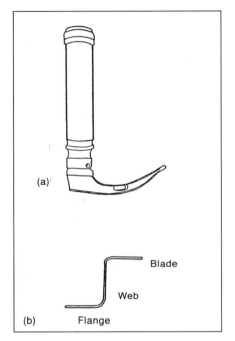

Figure 5.1. (a) Mackintosh curved-blade laryngoscope; (b) blade cross-section

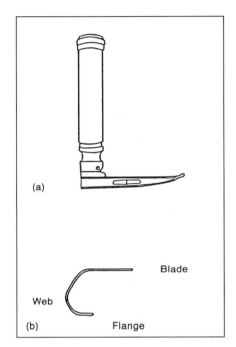

Figure 5.2. (a) Straight-blade laryngoscope; (b) blade cross-section

Endotracheal tubes

Endotracheal tubes come in a variety of designs, the most useful for resuscitation being the plain plastic tube. Uncuffed tubes are preferred up until puberty so as not to cause oedema at the cricoid ring. Red rubber tubes cause more local oedema if left in situ, and are used less often.

The Cole tube, with its shouldered tip, has been widely used in neonatal resuscitation. Its advantages were thought to be the lower rate of displacement into the bronchial tree, and a theoretical reduction in airway resistance because of the wider proximal tube diameter. It has been found that the shoulder may not only accentuate cricoid oedema but also cause turbulence, and therefore increase airway resistance. These tubes are therefore no longer recommended.

Estimating the appropriate size of an endotracheal tube is carried out as follows:

Internal diameter (mm) = (Age/4) + 4
Length (cm) = (Age/2) + 12 for an oral tube
Length (cm) = (Age/2) + 15 for a nasal tube

These formulae are appropriate for ages over 1 year. Neonates usually require a tube of internal diameter 3–3·5 mm, although pre-term infants may need one of diameter 2·5 mm. Another useful guideline is to use a tube of about the same diameter as the child's little finger, or of such a size that will just fit into the nostril.

35

Endotracheal tube introducers

A difficult intubation can be facilitated by the use of a stylet or introducer, placed through the lumen of the endotracheal tube. These are of two types: soft and flexible or firm and malleable. The former can be allowed to project out of the tip of the tube, as long as it is handled very gently. The latter is used to alter the shape of the tube, but can easily damage the tissues if allowed to protrude from the end.

Endotracheal tube connectors

In adults, the proximal end of the tube connectors is of standard size, based on the 15–22 mm system, ensuring that they can be connected to a standard self-inflating bag. The same standard Portex system exists for children, including neonates. However, many prefer to use smaller connectors in infants. The Mini-link system is based on diameters of 8·5 mm. Either system works well, but a resuscitation kit containing both can be confusing and dangerous. It is important that a clear decision between these is made so as to avoid this problem.

Magill's forceps

Magill's forceps are used to grasp an endotracheal tube, particularly one inserted through the nose, and pass it through the vocal cords. They are also suitable for removing foreign bodies in the upper airway under direct vision, and are designed to pass into the mouth with the handle at an angle so as not to obscure the view.

Tracheal suction catheters

These may be required after intubation to remove bronchial secretions or aspirated fluids. In general, the appropriate size in French gauge is numerically twice the internal diameter in millimetres, e.g. for an endotracheal tube size 3·0 mm the correct suction catheter is a French gauge 6.

Cricothyroidotomy cannulae and ventilation systems

Purpose-made cricothyroidotomy cannulae are available, usually in three sizes: 12-gauge for an adult, 14-gauge for a child, and 18-gauge for a baby. They are less liable to kinking than intravenous cannulae and have a flange for suturing or securing to the neck.

In an emergency a 14-gauge intravenous cannula can be inserted through the cricothyroid membrane, and oxygen insufflated at 2 l/min to provide some oxygenation (but no ventilation). A side hole can be cut in the oxygen tubing or a Y-connector can be placed between the cannula and the oxygen supply, to allow intermittent occlusion and achieve partial ventilation as described in Chapter 21.

EQUIPMENT FOR PROVIDING OXYGEN AND VENTILATION

The equipment for oxygenation and ventilation indicated in the box should be readily available.

Necessary equipment for oxygenation and ventilation

Oxygen source and masks for spontaneous breathing
Face masks (for artificial ventilation)
Self-inflating bags
T-piece and open-ended bag
Mechanical ventilators
Chest tubes
Gastric tubes

Oxygen source and masks for spontaneous breathing

A wall oxygen supply (at a pressure of 345 kPa or 50 p.s.i.) is provided in most resuscitation rooms. A flowmeter capable of delivering at least 15 l/min should be fitted.

In the older child, a "re-breather" mask with a reservoir bag should be used to supply a high concentration of oxygen. If a high concentration is not required, simple masks may be used. Nasal prongs are often well tolerated in pre-school age, but they cause drying of the airway, may cause nasal obstruction in infants, and provide an unreliable oxygen concentration. Venturi masks, head boxes, and oxygen tents are alternative devices, mainly used after initial treatment.

Younger children are more susceptible to the drying effect of a non-humidified oxygen supply.

Although the pre-term infant is vulnerable to retrolental fibroplasia caused by high-concentration oxygen, high concentrations should never be withheld for immediate resuscitation.

Face masks (for artificial ventilation)

Face masks for mouth-to-mask or bag–valve–mask ventilation in infants are of two main designs. Some masks conform to the anatomy of the child's face and have a low deadspace. Circular soft plastic masks give an excellent seal and are preferred by many. Children's masks should be clear to allow the child's colour or the presence of vomit to be seen.

The Laerdal pocket mask is a single-size clear plastic mask with an air-filled cushion rim designed for mouth-to-mask resuscitation. It can be supplied with a port for attaching to the oxygen supply and can be used in adults and children. By using it upside-down it may be used to ventilate an infant.

Self-inflating bags

Self-inflating bags come in three sizes: 240 ml, 500 ml, and 1600 ml. The two smaller sizes generally have a pressure-limiting valve set at 4·41 kPa (45 cmH$_2$O), which may (rarely) need to be overridden for high resistance/low compliance lungs, but which protects the normal lungs from inadvertent barotrauma. The patient end of the bag connects to a one-way valve of a fish-mouth or leaf-flap design. The opposite end has a connection to the oxygen supply, and to a reservoir attachment. The reservoir enables high oxygen concentrations to be delivered. Without it, it is difficult to supply more than 50% oxygen to the patient, whatever the fresh gas flow, whereas with it an inspired oxygen concentration of 98% can be achieved.

T-piece and open-ended bag

This equipment can only be used in children up to about 20 kg. It is used frequently by anaesthetists, but requires a "knack" to use it effectively. The open end of the bag is grasped by the ring and little fingers to regulate escape of the gas, while the rest of the hand squeezes the bag as shown in Figure 5.3. Nevertheless, in experienced hands, it does allow a reliable "feel" to the state of the lungs. It requires a reliable and controllable oxygen supply, and is totally ineffective if the supply fails. For this reason, self-inflating bags are generally preferred for initial resuscitation.

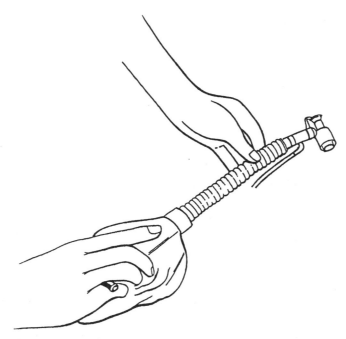

Figure 5.3. T-piece and open-ended bag

Mechanical ventilators

A detailed discussion of individual mechanical ventilators is beyond the scope of this book. Although clearly important in providing ventilation after initial resuscitation, they can give a false sense of security during inadequate or excessive ventilation. Continual re-evaluation is mandatory.

Chest tubes

These are included because haemopneumothorax may severely limit ventilation. They are described elsewhere.

Gastric tubes

Children are prone to air swallowing and vomiting. A gastric tube not only decompresses a distended stomach, but may significantly improve breathing. Withholding the procedure "to be kind to the child" may cause more distress than performing it.

PRACTICAL SKILLS

The following practical skills are described in detail in Chapter 21:

- Oropharyngeal airway insertion:
    small child
    older child.
- Nasopharyngeal airway insertion.
- Orotracheal intubation:
    infant/small child
    older child.
- Surgical airway:
    needle cricothyroidotomy
    surgical cricothyroidotomy.
- Ventilation without intubation:
    mouth-to-mask ventilation
    bag-and-mask ventilation.

The basic skills of head and neck positioning, chin lift and jaw thrust are discussed in Chapter 4.

Ventilation with a mechanical ventilator

A full description is beyond the scope of this book. In general, in small children, pressure-controlled ventilation is preferred. In this mode, gas flow is supplied to the child at a set pressure during inspiration, e.g. 1·50–1·96 kPa (15–20 cmH$_2$O). In the child with very stiff lungs, pressures of up to 2·94 kPa (30 cmH$_2$O) may be required. During expiration, a positive end-expiratory pressure (PEEP) is generally used, typically 294–490 Pa (3–5 cmH$_2$O). Pressure control partially compensates for any leak around the endotracheal cuff.

In the older child, controlled minute ventilation is a common mode of ventilation. The child receives a set volume of gas at a constant flow rate during inspiration, typically about 10 ml/kg.

In both the above modes, inspiratory and expiratory times are fixed. The inspiratory:expiratory (I:E) ratio is generally less than 1.

Other modes include synchronised intermittent mandatory volume (SIMV), pressure support, and continuous positive airway pressure (CPAP), but these are not discussed further.

PUTTING IT TOGETHER: AIRWAY-BREATHING MANAGEMENT

In order to respond urgently and yet retain thoroughness, effective emergency management demands a systematic, prioritised approach. Care can be structured into the four following phases.

Primary assessment

This consists of a rapid "physiological" examination to identify immediately life-threatening emergencies. It should be completed in less than a minute. It is prioritised as shown in the box.

> **Airway**
> **Breathing**
> **Circulation**
> **Disability (nervous system)**
> **Exposure**

From the respiratory viewpoint, do the following:

- Look, listen and feel for airway obstruction, respiratory arrest, depression, or distress.
- Assess the work of breathing.
- Count the respiratory rate.
- Listen for stridor and/or wheeze.
- Auscultate for breath sounds.
- Assess skin colour.

If a significant problem is identified, management should be started immediately. After appropriate interventions have been performed, primary assessment can be resumed or repeated.

Primary management (resuscitation)

During this phase, life-saving interventions are performed. These include such procedures as intubation, ventilation, cannulation, and fluid resuscitation. At the same time, oxygen is provided, vital signs are recorded, and essential monitoring is established.

From the respiratory viewpoint, do the following:

- Consider jaw- and neck-positioning manoeuvres.
- Administer oxygen.
- Consider suction and foreign body removal.
- Consider mask ventilation, and pharyngeal or tracheal intubation.
- Consider chest decompression.
- Consider needle cricothyroidotomy, if unable to oxygenate by alternative means.
- Initiate pulse oximetry and other monitoring at this time.

Secondary assessment

This consists of a thorough physical examination, together with appropriate investigations. Conventionally, examination is from head to toe, and represents an "anatomical" assessment. Before embarking on this phase, it is important that the resuscitative measures are fully under way.

From the respiratory viewpoint, do the following:

- Perform a detailed examination of the airway, neck, and chest.
- Identify any swelling, bruising, or wounds.
- Re-examine for symmetry of breath sounds and movement.
- Do not forget to inspect and listen to the back of the chest.

Secondary management

All other interventions are included in this phase.

If at any time the patient deteriorates, care returns to the primary assessment, and recycles through the system.

In the very sick or critically injured child, the primary assessment and management phases become integrally bound together. As a problem is identified, care shifts to the relevant intervention, before returning to the next part of the primary assessment. The simplified airway and breathing management protocol illustrates how this integration can be achieved.

Airway and breathing management protocol

Begin primary assessment.....
Assess the airway...
    If evidence of blunt trauma
        then protect the cervical spine from the outset
    If any evidence of obstruction and altered consciousness
        then optimise the head and neck positioning
        and administer oxygen
        and consider chin lift, jaw thrust, suction, foreign body removal
    If obstruction persists
        then consider oro- or nasopharyngeal airway
    If obstruction still persists
        then consider intubation
    If intubation impossible or unsuccessful
        then consider cricothyroidotomy
    If stridor but relatively alert
        then allow self-ventilation whenever possible
        and encourage oxygen but do not force to wear mask
        and do not force to lie down
        and do not inspect the airway (except as a definitive procedure under controlled conditions)
        and assemble expert team and equipment
Assess the breathing...
    If respiratory arrest or depression
        then administer oxygen by bag–valve–mask
        and consider intubation
    If sedative or paralysing drugs possible
        then administer reversal agent
    If respiratory distress or tachypnoea
        then administer oxygen
    If lateralised ventilatory deficit
        then consider haemopneumothorax and inhaled foreign body
        and consider lung consolidation, collapse, or pleural effusion
    If chest injury
        then consider tension pneumothorax and massive haemothorax
        and consider flail segment and open pneumothorax
    If evidence of tension pneumothorax
        then consider immediate needle decompression
        and follow up with chest drain
    If evidence of massive haemothorax
        then consider simultaneous chest drain
        and blood volume replacement
    If wheeze or crackles
        then consider asthma, bronchiolitis, pneumonia, and heart failure
        but remember inhaled foreign body as a possible cause
    If evidence of acute severe asthma
        then consider inhaled or intravenous β-agonists
        and consider intravenous steroids and aminophylline
    If evidence of heart failure
        then consider frusemide and inotropes
Continue the primary assessment....
    .... proceed to assess the circulation and nervous system
    If deteriorating from whatever cause
        then reassess the airway and breathing
        and be prepared to intubate and ventilate

6

The management of cardiac arrest

Cardiac arrest has occurred when there are no palpable central pulses. Before any specific therapy is started effective basic life support must be established as described in Chapter 4. Three cardiac arrest rhythms will be discussed in this chapter:

1. Asystole.
2. Ventricular fibrillation.
3. Electromechanical dissociation.

ASYSTOLE

This is the most common arrest rhythm in children, because the response of the young heart to prolonged severe hypoxia and acidosis is progressive bradycardia leading to asystole.

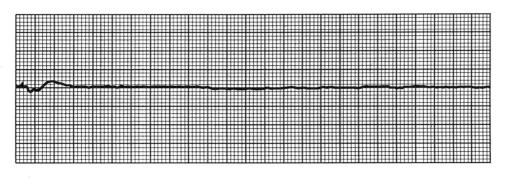

Figure 6.1. Asystole

The ECG will distinguish asystole from ventricular fibrillation and electromechanical dissociation (Figure 6.1). The ECG appearance of ventricular asystole is an almost straight line; occasionally P waves are seen. Check that the appearance is not caused by an artefact, e.g. a loose wire or disconnected electrode. Turn up the gain on the ECG monitor.

Drugs in asystole

Before the administration of any drug the patient must be receiving continuous and effective basic life support, have a patent airway, and be adequately ventilated with high-concentration oxygen.

The protocol for drug use in asystole is shown in Figure 6.2.

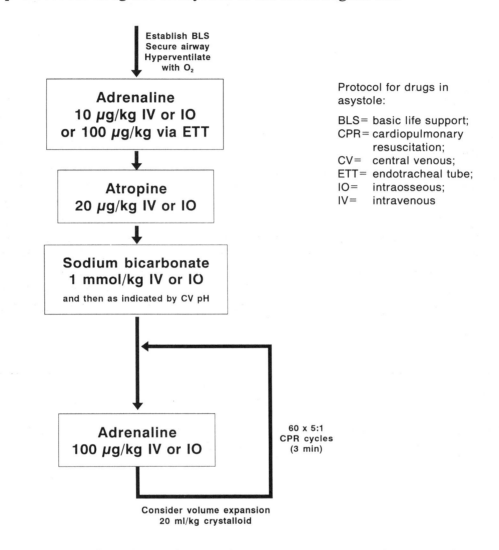

Figure 6.2. Protocol for drugs in asystole. BLS=basic life support; CPR=cardiopulmonary resuscitation; CV=central venous; ETT=endotracheal tube; IO=intraosseous; IV=intravenous

Adrenaline

Adrenaline is the first-line drug for asystole. The initial intravenous dose is 10 μg/kg (0·1 ml of 1:10 000 solution). This is best given through a central line, but if one is not in place it may be given through a peripheral or intraosseous line followed by a normal (or physiological) saline flush (2–5 ml). If there is no vascular access, the endotracheal tube can be used. Ten times the intravenous dose (i.e. 100 μg/kg) should be given via this route. The drug should be injected quickly down a narrow-bore suction catheter beyond the tracheal end of the endotracheal tube and then flushed in with 1 or 2 ml normal (physiological) saline. In patients with pulmonary disease or prolonged asystole, pulmonary oedema and intrapulmonary shunting may make the endotracheal route less effective. If there has been no clinical effect, further doses should be given intravenously as soon as venous access has been secured.

Atropine

Atropine should be given intravenously (0·02 mg/kg) or intratracheally (0·04 mg/kg). There is no clear evidence that atropine is useful in cardiac arrest, but it is used to counteract vagal stimulation and to increase cardiac conductivity.

Sodium bicarbonate

Children with asystole are usually profoundly acidotic as their cardiac arrest has usually been preceded by respiratory arrest or shock. The efficacy of adrenaline is reduced in acidosis and therefore sodium bicarbonate (1 mmol/kg) should precede further doses of adrenaline.

The use of bicarbonate in cardiac arrest is now more sparing than in the past. Sodium bicarbonate is an irritant and hyperosmolar drug which contains a high concentration of sodium. It produces carbon dioxide which may cause hypercapnia in the unventilated patient. In addition it causes intracellular acidosis despite temporarily raising the intravascular pH. In ventilated children, however, this excess carbon dioxide can be removed by hyperventilation. The dose for children is 1 mmol/kg (8·4% solution 1 ml/kg). In neonates the 8·4% solution should be diluted to 4·2%. Central venous pH should be used to guide the use of further boluses of sodium bicarbonate. Arterial blood gas monitoring is unhelpful as a guide to bicarbonate use in cardiac arrest because arterial pH is unlikely to reflect tissue pH.

- Bicarbonate must not be given in the same intravenous line as calcium because precipitation will occur
- Sodium bicarbonate inactivates adrenaline and dopamine, and therefore the line must be flushed with saline if these drugs are subsequently given
- Bicarbonate may not be given by the intratracheal route

Continuing the protocol

A second bolus of adrenaline (at a dose of ten times the first) should be given if spontaneous cardiac output has not returned. At this stage expansion of the circulating volume should be considered, and 20 ml/kg of crystalloid (such as normal (physiological) saline or Ringer's lactate) should be used to achieve this. This is because the arrest may have been precipitated by hypovolaemia and, even if it were not, increasing the preload may prove beneficial.

If there is still no response, continue to administer adrenaline 100 µg/kg every 3 minutes (60 × 5:1 CPR cycles). A continuous infusion of adrenaline at 2 µg/kg/min may be tried as an alternative to this. Evidence suggests that the outcome of asystole in childhood is very poor if there is no response to the second dose of adrenaline.

Check that the intravenous line is still patent. Try a central venous line if drugs do not seem to be effective through a peripheral line.

There is no evidence that calcium is helpful in asystole. In fact, calcium can be detrimental, causing coronary artery spasm, and should only be used to treat documented hypocalcaemia, hyperkalaemia, or hypermagnesaemia.

VENTRICULAR FIBRILLATION

The ECG for ventricular fibrillation is shown in Figure 6.3.

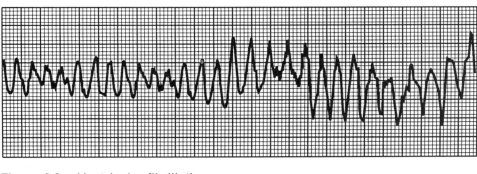

Figure 6.3. Ventricular fibrillation

This arrhythmia is uncommon in children but should be sought in those who are recovering from hypothermia, those poisoned by tricyclic antidepressants, and those with cardiac disease. The protocol for ventricular fibrillation is shown in Figure 6.4.

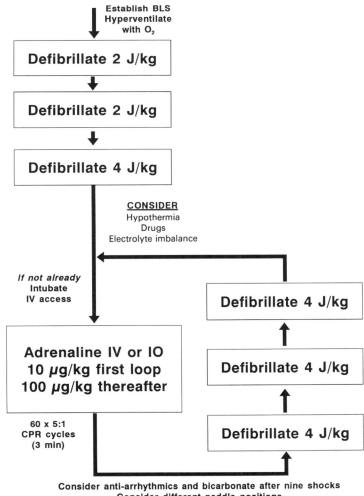

Figure 6.4. Protocol for ventricular fibrillation

46

Asynchronous electrical defibrillation should be carried out immediately. There is no place for a precordial thump in children. Paediatric paddles (4·5 cm) should be used for children under 10 kg. One electrode is placed over the apex in the mid-axillary line, whilst the other is put immediately below the clavicle just to the right of the sternum. If only adult paddles are available for an infant under 10 kg, one may be placed on the infant's back and one over the left lower part of the chest at the front.

The initial two shocks should be given at 2 J/kg. If these two attempts are unsuccessful the third attempt should be at 4 J/kg. If three shocks fail to produce defibrillation, the patient should be hyperventilated (to increase pH), given adrenaline, either 10 µg/kg intravenously or intraosseously or 100 µg/kg via the tracheal route, and three further shocks (4 J/kg) given. If this is ineffective, the adrenaline dose should be increased to 100 µg/kg intravenously or intraosseously followed by three further shocks 1 minute later.

The underlying cause of the arrhythmia should be considered. If ventricular fibrillation is due to hypothermia then defibrillation may be resistant until core temperature is increased. Active rewarming should be commenced. If drug overdose underlies the fibrillation, then specific anti-arrhythmic agents may be needed.

The use of an alkylating agent such as sodium bicarbonate (1 mmol/kg intravenously or intraosseously) or an anti-arrhythmic agent such as lignocaine (1 mg/kg intravenously or intraosseously) should also be considered. Lignocaine may be given intratracheally at twice the usual intravenous dose. There is little evidence about the usefulness of the anti-arrhythmic agent bretyllium tosylate in children, but it may be given in a dose of 5 mg/kg at this stage in children over 12 years old.

If there is still resistance to defibrillation different paddle positions or another defibrillator may be tried.

ELECTROMECHANICAL DISSOCIATION

This is the absence of a palpable pulse despite the presence of recognisable complexes on the ECG monitor. The most common cause in childhood is profound shock which makes the pulse difficult to feel. The protocol for electromechanical dissociation is shown in Figure 6.5. Electromechanical dissociation should be treated with rapid volume expansion of crystalloid or colloid (20 ml/kg) and adrenaline (10 µg/kg) after basic life support, intubation, and ventilation have been established. If there is no return of a palpable pulse, the next adrenaline dose should be 100 µg/kg.

Throughout management the underlying cause should be sought. As mentioned above, hypovolaemia is the most common cause in childhood. However, tension pneumothorax and cardiac tamponade should also be considered in the trauma patient. Rarely, pulmonary embolus may be the cause. In other patients electrolyte disturbance may underlie electromechanical dissociation, and in this group the use of calcium chloride (10–30 mg/kg intravenously) should be considered (see Appendix B). This drug should be given slowly into a peripheral vein. Calcium may have serious toxic effects such as bradycardia, coronary artery spasms, and myocardial irritability. It is also implicated as a mediator of post-ischaemic cellular damage. It can cause severe local tissue damage if extravasated into tissues.

While treatable causes are being excluded persistent electromechanical dissociation should be treated like asystole.

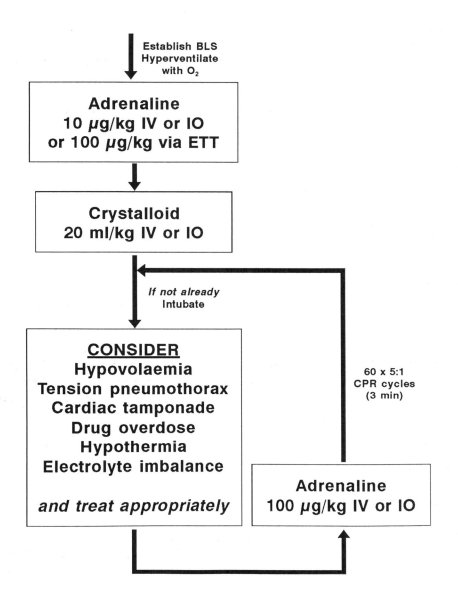

Figure 6.5. Protocol for electromechanical dissociation

POST-RESUSCITATION MANAGEMENT

Once spontaneous cardiac output has been established, frequent clinical reassessment must be carried out to detect deterioration or improvement with therapy. All patients should be monitored for the following:

- Pulse rate and rhythm.
- Oxygen saturation.
- Core temperature.
- Skin temperature.
- Blood pressure.
- Urine output.
- Arterial pH and gases.

Additionally some patients will require:

- CO_2 monitoring.
- Invasive BP monitoring.

48

- Central venous pressure monitoring.
- Intracranial pressure monitoring.

The investigation shown in the box should be performed immediately following successful resuscitation:

Investigation

- Chest radiograph
- Twelve-lead ECG
- Arterial and central venous blood gases
- Haemoglobin, haematocrit, and platelets
- Group and save serum for cross-match
- Na^+, K^+, urea, and creatinine concentrations
- Clotting screen
- Blood glucose
- Liver function tests

Often children who have been resuscitated from cardiac arrest die hours or days later from multisystem organ failure. In addition to the cellular and homoeostatic abnormalities that occur during the preceding illness, and during the arrest itself, cellular damage continues after spontaneous circulation has been restored. This is called reperfusion injury and is caused by the following:

- Depletion of ATP.
- Entry of calcium into cells.
- Free fatty acid metabolism activation.
- Free oxygen radical production.

Post-resuscitation management aims to achieve and maintain homoeostasis in order to optimise the chances of recovery. Management should be directed in a systematic way.

Airway and breathing

Most recently resuscitated patients will have an impaired conscious level or depressed gag reflex. These children should remain intubated, and should be ventilated with a fractional concentration of inspired oxygen (F_{IO_2}) which is sufficient to keep oxygen saturation above 95%; other ventilation parameters should be set to keep blood gases as normal as possible.

Circulation

Following cardiac arrest from any cause there will usually be poor cardiac output. This may be due to any combination of the following factors:

- Underlying cardiac abnormality.
- Effects on myocardium of hypoxia, acidosis, and toxins, preceding and during arrest.
- Continuing acid–base or electrolyte disturbance.
- Hypovolaemia.

The following steps should be taken if there are signs of poor perfusion:

- Assess cardiac output clinically.
- Ensure normal arterial pH and oxygenation.
- Identify and start to correct electrolyte abnormality or hypoglycaemia.
- Infuse crystalloid or colloid 20 ml/kg and reassess cardiac output clinically.

At this stage, there may be a need for:

- Further circulatory expansion.
- Inotropic drug support of the myocardium.
- Vasodilatation of the circulatory system.

A central venous pressure line will give useful information about systemic venous pressure which will assist in the decisions about fluid infusion or inotropic support. The central venous pressure measures right ventricular function and the effect of venous return on preload.

The central venous pressure is best used in assessing the response to a fluid challenge. In hypovolaemic patients, central venous pressure alters little with a fluid bolus, but in euvolaemia or hypervolaemia it shows a sustained rise. Further details on inotropic and vasodilator drugs will be found in Chapter 10.

Kidney

It is important both to maximise renal blood flow and to maintain renal tubular patency by maintaining urine flow. To achieve this the following are necessary:

- Maintenance of good oxygenation.
- Maintenance of good circulation using inotropes or fluids as required.
- Judicious use of diuretics (e.g. frusemide 1 mg/kg) to maintain urine output at or above 1 ml/kg/kg.
- Monitoring and normalisation of electrolytes (Na^+ and K^+) and acid–base balance in blood and urine.

Liver

Hepatic cellular damage can become manifest up to 24 hours following an arrest. Among other things coagulation factors can become depleted, and bleeding may be worsened by concomitant, ischaemia-induced, intravascular coagulopathy. The following should be done: monitoring of clotting, and correction as indicated.

Brain

The aim of therapy is to protect the brain from further (secondary) damage. To achieve this the cerebral blood flow must be maintained, normal cellular homoeostasis must be achieved, and cerebral metabolic needs must be reduced.

Adequate cerebral blood flow can only be achieved if the cerebral perfusion pressure (*mean arterial pressure − intracranial pressure*) is kept about 50 mmHg. Cellular homoeostasis is helped by normalisation of acid–base and electrolyte balances. Cerebral metabolic needs can be reduced by sedating the child and by controlling convulsions. Although barbiturate coma does reduce cerebral metabolism, it has not been shown to improve neurological outcome.

Practical steps to minimise secondary brain injury are:

- Maintenance of good oxygenation.
- Maintenance of good circulation using inotropes or fluids as required.
- Monitoring and normalisation of electrolytes (Na^+ and K^+) and acid–base balance.
- Normalisation of blood glucose.
- Normalisation of body temperature.
- Maintenance of adequate analgaesia and sedation.
- Reduction of intracranial pressure (see Chapter 17).

Hypothermia and hypoglycaemia

Hypothermia

Sick or injured children become cold easily; therefore they should either be kept covered with blankets or should be placed under an infrared heater. The rectal temperature should be monitored.

Hypoglycaemia

All children, and most particularly infants, have poor glycogen stores and may become hypoglycaemic when seriously ill. Blood sugar must be checked and dextrose 10% (in infants) or 25% (in older children) given if indicated.

WHEN TO STOP RESUSCITATION

If there have been no detectable signs of cardiac output, and there has been no evidence of cerebral activity despite 30 minutes of cardiopulmonary resuscitation, it is reasonable to stop resuscitation. The decision will be taken by the team leader.

Exceptions to this rule include the hypothermic child (in whom resuscitation must continue until the patient has a core temperature of at least 32°C) and children who have taken overdoses of cerebral depressant drugs such as phenobarbitone. In both these cases prolonged resuscitation attempts will be necessary.

7

Resuscitation of the newborn

RELEVANT PHYSIOLOGY

After delivery of a healthy term baby the first breath usually occurs within 60 seconds of the umbilical cord being clamped. Clamping leads to the onset of asphyxia which is the major stimulant to the start of respiration. Physical stimuli, e.g. cold air or physical discomfort, help provoke respiratory efforts. Squeezing of the baby through the maternal pelvis generates a positive pressure around the baby's chest of 50 cmH$_2$O (4·9 kPa). In a vigorous baby unaffected by intra partum asphyxia, drugs, or prematurity, the first spontaneous breath generates a negative pressure of between -40 and -100 cmH$_2$O ($-3·9$ and $-9·8$ kPa). This is necessary to overcome the viscosity of fluid filling the airways, the surface tension in the fluid-filled lungs, and the elastic recoil and resistance of the chest wall, lungs, and airways. The pressure necessary at this time is 10–15 times greater than that needed for later breathing when the lungs are fully aerated.

Babies born by caesarean section are less likely to form a functional residual capacity with the first breath than if they had been born vaginally.

The fluid that fills the lungs usually clears by the age of 1 hour and approximately 35 ml will drain from the mouth of a baby born vaginally at term. The rest will be absorbed by the lung capillaries and lymphatics as they open up. Prolonged high pressure on expiration, i.e. by crying, helps this process.

Surfactant (which is 85% lipid) is made by the type II (granular) pneumocytes in the alveolar epithelium. Surfactant reduces alveolar surface tension and prevents alveolar collapse on expiration. Production of surfactant is reduced if the temperature falls below 35°C, if there is hypoxia, or if the pH drops below 7·25. Type II pneumocytes and surfactant can be demonstrated in the fetal lung at 20 weeks' gestation. There is initially a slow increase in production until a surge occurs at 30–34 weeks. Surfactant is released at birth due to ventilation and distension of the alveoli. The half-life of surfactant once released is approximately 12 hours.

If in a particular baby there is a lack of surfactant, respiratory work is increased in an effort to get adequate alveolar ventilation. Intrapulmonary shunting occurs past partially collapsed or fully collapsed alveoli leading to hypoxia and a drop in pH.

PRACTICAL ASPECTS OF NEONATAL RESUSCITATION

(*Note that this section assumes that there is no suspicion of the meconium aspiration syndrome. For details on special aspects of resuscitation following meconium aspiration see section at the end of this chapter.*)

Apgar score (Table 7.1)

The Apgar scoring system was developed as a tool to indicate the baby's condition at birth. Five physical signs are examined and the score computed at 1 and 5 minutes after birth.

Table 7.1. Apgar scoring

Score	Heart rate	Respirations	Muscle tone	Reflex irritability (catheter in nares)	Colour
0	Absent	Absent	Limp	No response	Blue or pale
1	Slow (<100/min)	Slow, irregular	Some flexion	Grimace	Pink body with blue extremities
2	>100/min	Good, crying	Active motion	Cough or sneeze	Completely pink

Although the Apgar score is useful for those experienced in its use, treatment should not be delayed while it is computed. Need for resuscitation should therefore be assessed by examining *colour*, *heart rate* (by auscultation), and *respiratory effort*; the baby may then be broadly categorised into one of four groups, as follows (Table 7.2).

Healthy
Pink and crying lustily with a heart rate greater than 100/min. These babies need no further treatment.

Primary apnoea
Heart rate greater than 80/min, baby cyanosed with some tone, and possibly some response to stimulation (fetal pH likely to be >7.25). These babies may begin to breathe spontaneously and a short wait (not >1 min) with gentle stimulation and "blow by" oxygen is acceptable initially.

Terminal apnoea
Heart rate less than 80/min, baby pale, floppy, and apnoeic (fetal pH likely to be <7.25). Bag-and-mask ventilation is necessary, followed by intubation if there is no rapid response. These babies will not breathe without help.

Fresh stillbirth
Apnoeic, pale, floppy, and asystolic. Full cardiopulmonary resuscitation, including cardiac compression and possibly drug administration, is required.

Table 7.2. Initial resuscitation of a newborn

Category	Initial findings	Action
Healthy	Pink HR >100 Good respiratory effort	Dry Keep warm Give to mother
Primary apnoea	Blue HR >80 Apnoeic or gasping	Gentle suction O_2 by mask ?Bag/mask ventilation ← 1 min
Terminal apnoea	White Heart rate <80 Apnoeic	Gentle suction Bag/mask ventilation ?Intubation
Fresh stillbirth	White Asystolic Apnoeic	Intubation Cardiac compression ?Drugs

Temperature control

Newborns become cold very quickly; a cold baby has an increased O_2 consumption, and a propensity to hypoglycaemia and acidosis. The delivery should take place in a warm room and, if possible, an overhead heater should be switched on. The baby should also be dried immediately to prevent evaporative heat loss and, if no intervention is required, it should be wrapped in a warm blanket.

Suction

As a general rule, only soft suction catheters should be used with a maximum negative pressure of 13·3 kPa (100 mmHg). Healthy babies will clear their own secretions and do not need suction. The others will benefit from suction of the external nares and the mouth, but deep pharyngeal suction should be avoided as vagal stimulation resulting in bradycardia or laryngospasm may occur (see "Meconium aspiration", later).

Oxygen

This is the most useful drug in resuscitation at birth. Oxygen 100% may safely be given even to pre-term babies for short periods.

Bag/mask ventilation

A mask that is big enough to cover the face from the bridge of the nose to below the mouth should be chosen. Most people prefer the transparent circular type. The reservoir bag should have a volume of 500 ml as this allows a sustained initial breath to be performed in order to inflate the fetal lung. There should be a blow-off valve which operates at 30–40 cmH$_2$O (2·9–3·9 kPa), but it should be possible to override this if a greater inflation pressure is necessary. The bag should be connected to an oxygen supply and must have a reservoir to allow the delivery of high concentrations of oxygen.

Tracheal intubation

This will be necessary if a baby with primary apnoea does not response promptly to bag-mask ventilation, or for babies in secondary apnoea or asystole. Pre-term babies are more likely to require intubation. The advantage of the tracheal tube is that it allows more effective inflation of the fetal lung. Conversely barotrauma, such as pneumothorax, is more likely once it is in place.

The technique of intubation is the same as for infants and is described in Chapter 21. A normal, full-term infant usually needs a 3·00 mm endotracheal tube, but 2·5 and 3·5 mm tubes should also be available. The first inflation should be held for 2–3 seconds. A rate of 30–40 breaths/min should then be maintained. If there are still poor chest movements, the pressure can be increased to 3·9 kPa (40 cmH$_2$O).

Cardiac compression

Cardiac compression must be started if the heart rate is below 80/min. The most efficient way of doing this in a neonate is to encircle the chest with both hands, so that the fingers lie behind the baby and the thumbs are apposed over the mid-sternum. The sternum should be depressed at a rate of 120/min. This technique gives the optimum cardiac output and blood pressure. Give three chest compressions for each inhalation.

Drugs

If a baby has failed to increase his or her heart rate, and is still pale or blue after adequate ventilation with 100% oxygen and chest compressions:

1. Give 10 µg/kg adrenaline intravenously or intratracheally.
2. Give 1 mmol/kg of $NaHCO_3$ intravenously (use 4·2% solution).
3. Further doses of adrenaline 10–30 µg/kg may be given every 3–5 minutes if there is no response.

Actions in event of poor initial response to resuscitation

1. Check for technical fault
   (a) Is oxygen connected?
   (b) Is endotracheal tube in the trachea? Auscultate chest and observe chest movement.
   (c) Is endotracheal tube too far down in a bronchus? Listen to both sides of chest for unequal air entry.
   (d) Is endotracheal tube blocked?
   If any doubt remains about the positioning or patency of the endotracheal tube it should be removed and replaced by a fresh tube.
2. Does the baby have a pneumothorax? Auscultate the chest for asymmetry of breath sounds; feel for a displaced cardiac apex and trachea. A cold light source can be used to trans-illuminate the chest – a pneumothorax may show as a hyper-illuminating area. If a tension pneumothorax is thought to be present clinically, a 21-gauge butterfly needle should be inserted through the second intercostal space in the mid-clavicular line. The end of the butterfly tube should be in a gallipot under saline. If a pneumothorax is present, air bubbles will be seen in the saline, and the baby will improve as pneumothorax is no longer under tension. A confirmatory radiograph can now be done and a chest drain inserted.
3. Does the baby have evolving lung disease, such as respiratory distress syndrome or congenital pneumonia? If the lungs are stiff to ventilate, increased frequency and pressure of ventilation should be tried.
4. Is the baby suffering from the effects of maternal opiate sedation? This may be the case if the baby has become pink with a good heart rate, but there is no respiratory effort when ventilation is stopped. If respiratory depressant effects are suspected the baby should be given naloxone 10 µg/kg intravenously. The effects of this drug are very short acting, and a second dose or an infusion may be necessary.
5. Does the baby have a congenital abnormality obstructing respiration, such as a diaphragmatic hernia? This can be diagnosed on a chest radiograph, but only supportive treatment is feasible until the child is transferred to a neonatal surgical unit.
6. Is there severe anaemia? If there was fetal blood loss during delivery, then 4·5% albumin 20 ml/kg, other colloid, or non-cross-matched O-negative blood should be given immediately. A blood transfusion cross-matched with mother's and baby's blood should be given as soon as possible.
   Some babies may be severely anaemic from haemolytic disease and are not hypovolaemic. These babies require exchange transfusion with packed red blood cells. They may also have bilateral pleural effusions which require drainage.
7. Does the baby have congenital cyanotic heart disease? If the baby is being adequately ventilated and has a good heart rate and peripheral perfusion, but remains cyanosed, then a diagnosis of congenital heart disease may be considered (see Chapter 10).

Note: during the process of a prolonged resuscitation, hypoglycaemia should be sought and treated with 10% dextrose 5 ml/kg intravenously.

Prematurity

The more pre-term an infant is, the more likely it is that spontaneous respiratory efforts will not be adequate. One has to anticipate that babies born before 32 weeks will need some help to establish prompt ventilation and there is evidence to suggest that the more quickly the baby becomes pink with adequate breathing the less likelihood there is of subsequent hyaline membrane disease.

Pre-term babies are likely to be deficient in surfactant and may need relatively higher inflation pressures than term babies. It is appropriate to start resuscitating such a baby with a pressure of 2·0–2·5 kPa (20–25 cmH$_2$O) but to increase this if resuscitation does not produce satisfactory chest wall movements.

Fresh stillbirth

If fetal monitors showed signs of life shortly before delivery, it is justifiable to carry out full cardiopulmonary resuscitation on fresh stillbirths. In some babies the eventual outcome will be extremely good. When full resuscitation has been embarked upon, it may be difficult to know when to stop. Published data suggest that if there is still no sign of life whatsoever after 10 minutes, then very few babies will survive and moreover those who do will have cerebral palsy. If the heart rate responds to resuscitation, but there is no sustained spontaneous respiration after 30 minutes, then the outlook is equally poor.

Resuscitation of the newborn in the accident and emergency department

Most newborn resuscitation procedures take place in the controlled environment of the delivery room or of the neonatal intensive care unit. Under these circumstances the maternal history is readily available. However, if an infant is brought to the accident and emergency department for resuscitation, delivery has often been sudden and unexpected, and little history is available. The following historical points should be sought rapidly, as they may influence the type of resuscitation needed:

- Was there an ante-partum haemorrhage? If so the baby may be expected to be severely asphyxiated.
- Is the infant expected to be pre-term? Resuscitation will almost certainly be required.
- Has the cord been clamped adequately? If not the baby may be hypovolaemic from blood loss.
- Is the birth a singleton? If twins are expected two resuscitations may be necessary.
- Is there a history of meconium in the amniotic fluid? Resuscitation may need to include tracheal suction.

In addition to resuscitation equipment for infants referred to in previous chapters, the following will be necessities for resuscitation of the newborn in the accident and emergency department:

1. Radiant warmer.
2. Warmed towels for drying infant.
3. Mechanical suction device.
4. Umbilical catheter (French 5-gauge).
5. Umbilical cord tie and scalpel.

MECONIUM ASPIRATION

Pathophysiology

Hypoxia in a near-term fetus (37 weeks or more) leads to gut vessel vasoconstriction, an increase in peristalsis, and relaxation of the sphincters. This in turn leads to the passing of meconium in utero. In addition fetal hypoxia causes the normal rapid (30–70/min) shallow fetal respirations to stop completely, and the fetus becomes apnoeic for a period of time. Continuation of asphyxia leads to deep gasping respirations in utero with aspiration of amniotic fluid and the meconium within it.

Once meconium gets into the lungs it causes problems in several different ways. There can be complete obstruction of an airway leading to collapse of a lung lobe. There can be partial obstruction of an airway leading to a ball valve effect and over-distension, perhaps leading to pulmonary interstitial emphysema and pneumothorax. Meconium, which is irritant but sterile, can also lead to chemical pneumonitis and can increase the risks of secondary lung infection.

In addition, the asphyxial insult can lead to persistent pulmonary hypertension, cerebral ischaemia, myocardial ischaemia, and renal ischaemia.

Special aspects of resuscitation

If meconium aspiration is suspected it is advisable to suction the pharynx after delivery of the baby's head. If the baby shows depression of respiratory effort, the pharynx should be sucked out before the baby is either encouraged to breathe or given artificial respiratory support. Some advise that the baby's chest should be held to prevent gasping while suction is being carried out.

If there is meconium in the mouth, inspect the larynx. Intubate the baby if meconium is present at this level so as to allow suctioning below the vocal cords. Meconium will not be removed by a fine suction catheter passed through an endotracheal tube. Therefore, suction is applied directly to the endotracheal tube and the tube is slowly withdrawn. The infant is then reintubated with a clean tube and the procedure repeated. When suctioning the newborn trachea in this way, negative pressure should not exceed $-100\,\text{mmHg}$ ($-9.8\,\text{kPa}$), and suction should be brief and intermittent.

PART

III

THE SERIOUSLY ILL CHILD

8

Respiratory emergencies

Disorders of the respiratory tract are the most common illnesses of childhood. They are the most frequent reason for children to be seen by their general practitioner and they account for 30–40% of acute medical admissions to hospital in children. Despite advances in the management of respiratory illnesses, they still result in over 450 deaths in children between the ages of 4 weeks and 14 years in England and Wales each year: over 70% of these deaths are in children less than 12 months old.

Many respiratory illnesses are self-limiting minor infections, but others present as potentially life-threatening emergencies. In these, accurate diagnosis and prompt initiation of appropriate treatment are essential if unnecessary morbidity and mortality are to be avoided.

SUSCEPTIBILITY OF CHILDREN TO SEVERE RESPIRATORY ILLNESS

The pattern of severe respiratory illness in children is different from that in adults. These variations reflect important differences in the immune status, and the structure and function of the lungs and chest wall of children and adults.

- Children, and particularly infants, are *susceptible to infection* with many organisms to which adults have acquired immunity.
- The upper and the lower *airways in children are smaller*, and are more easily obstructed by mucosal swelling, secretions, or a foreign body. Airway resistance is inversely proportional to the fourth power of the radius of the airway: a reduction in the radius by a half causes a sixteenfold increase in airway resistance. Thus, 1 mm of mucosal oedema in an infant's trachea of 5 mm diameter results in a much greater increase in resistance than the same degree of oedema in the trachea of 10 mm diameter.
- The *thoracic cage* of young children is much more compliant than that of adults. When there is airway obstruction and increased inspiratory effort, this increased compliance results in marked chest wall recession and a reduction in the efficiency of breathing.
- The *respiratory muscles* of young children are relatively inefficient. In infancy, the diaphragm is the principal respiratory muscle, and the intercostal and accessory muscles make relatively little contribution. Respiratory muscle fatigue can develop rapidly and result in respiratory failure and apnoea.

ASSESSMENT OF RESPIRATORY EMERGENCIES IN CHILDHOOD

The respiratory illnesses in children that present most commonly as emergencies are as follows:

- Upper airway obstruction, e.g. croup, epiglottitis.
- Lower airway obstruction, asthma, bronchiolitis.
- Pneumonia.

Although all of these diseases result in respiratory distress, it is possible to distinguish between them with a careful history and clinical examination. As the appropriate treatment for each of these disorders is quite specific, it is imperative that the correct diagnosis of the cause of the respiratory distress is made.

History

Important symptoms are summarised in Table 8.1.

Table 8.1. Symptoms in respiratory emergencies

Symptom	Comment
Breathlessness	? At rest
	? When walking upstairs
	? When talking
	? When sleeping (in older children)
	? When feeding (in infants)
Cough	Barking or seal-like in croup
	Dry and wheezy in bronchiolitis
Noisy breathing	Stridor, mainly inspiratory, due to narrowing of trachea or larynx
	Wheezy, mainly expiratory, due to more distal obstruction in respiratory tree
Hoarseness	Vocal cord (vocal fold) involvement
Drooling and inability to drink	Epiglottitis
Abdominal pain	Sometimes present in pneumonia
Meningism	Sometimes present in pneumonia

High fever, lethargy, and anorexia are common in children with respiratory infections.

Examination

Careful inspection of the child's respiratory pattern, posture, and behaviour is often the most informative part of the physical examination, particularly in younger children. Remember that diseases other than respiratory illnesses can produce many of these signs. For example, deep rapid respirations may indicate metabolic acidosis or salicylate poisoning. It can be difficult to distinguish between respiratory disease and congenital heart disease in the young child. Both give rise to tachypnoea, tachycardia, and cyanosis. Congenital heart disease is more likely if there is evidence of heart failure such as liver enlargement or a triple cardiac rhythm. Cardiac murmurs or an irregular pulse also suggest primary heart disease.

Further useful information about the severity of the illness may be provided by measurement of the *oxygen saturation* levels with a pulse oximeter. *Arterial blood gases* are needed if there is evidence of respiratory or circulatory failure. In children over the age of 5 years with asthma, measurement of the *peak expiratory flow rate* should be a routine part of the initial assessment. A *chest radiograph* is often helpful, particularly in the young infant where physical signs may be difficult to interpret.

UPPER AIRWAY OBSTRUCTION

Obstruction of the upper airway (larynx and trachea) is potentially life threatening. As mentioned above, the small cross-sectional area of the upper airway renders the young child particularly vulnerable to obstruction by oedema, secretions, or an inhaled foreign body.

The cardinal feature of upper airway obstruction is *stridor*, which is heard predominantly during inspiration, but which may also be audible in expiration. Like the wheeze in asthma, the intensity of the stridor does not indicate the severity of the obstruction. In addition to the stridor, there may be *hoarseness* due to swelling of the vocal cords (vocal folds), and a *barking* or *seal-like cough*. The severity of obstruction is best assessed by the degree of sternal and subcostal *recession*, and the respiratory and heart rate. Increasing *agitation* or *drowsiness*, or central *cyanosis*, indicates severe hypoxaemia and the need for urgent intervention.

Differential diagnosis of acute upper airway obstruction

Most cases of upper airway obstruction in children are the result of infection, but inhalation of a foreign body or hot gases (house fires), angioneurotic oedema, and trauma can all result in such obstruction.

Incidence	Diagnoses
Very common	Croup – viral laryngotracheitis
Common	Croup – recurrent or spasmodic croup
Uncommon	Epiglottitis
	Laryngeal foreign body
Rare	Croup – bacterial tracheitis
	Diphtheria
	Retropharyngeal abscess
	Infectious mononucleosis
	Angioneurotic oedema
	Inhalation of hot gases
	Trauma

Croup

Croup is defined as an acute clinical syndrome with inspiratory stridor, a barking cough, hoarseness, and variable degrees of respiratory distress. This definition embraces several distinct disorders. Acute *viral laryngotracheobronchitis (viral croup)* is the most common form of croup and accounts for over 95% of laryngotracheal infections. Parainfluenza viruses are the most common pathogens but other respiratory viruses, such as respiratory syncytial virus and adenoviruses, produce a similar clinical picture. The peak incidence of viral croup is in the second year of life, and most hospital admissions are in children aged between 6 months and 5 years. The typical features of a barking cough, harsh stridor, and hoarseness are usually preceded by fever and coryza for 1–3 days. The symptoms often start, and are worse, at night. Many children have stridor and a mild fever (<38·5°C), with little or no respiratory difficulty. If tracheal narrowing is minor, stridor will be present only when the child hyperventilates or is upset. As the narrowing progresses, the stridor becomes both inspiratory and expiratory, and is present even when the child is at rest. Some children, and particularly those below the age of 3 years, develop the features of increasing obstruction and hypoxaemia.

Some children have repeated episodes of croup without preceding fever and coryza. The symptoms are often of sudden onset at night, and often persist for only a few hours. This *recurrent* or *spasmodic croup* is often associated with atopic disease (asthma, eczema, hay fever). The episodes can be severe, but are more commonly self-limiting.

Bacterial tracheitis, or *pseudomembranous croup*, is an uncommon, but life-threatening, form of croup. Infection of the tracheal mucosa with *Staphylococcus aureus*, streptococci or *Haemophilus influenzae B* results in copious, purulent secretions and mucosal necrosis. The child appears toxic with a high fever and the signs of progressive upper airway obstruction. The croupy cough and the absence of drooling help distinguish this condition from epiglottitis. Over 80% of children with this illness need intubation and ventilatory support to maintain an adequate airway, as well as intravenous antibiotics (combination of ampicillin and flucloxacillin, or ceftazidine).

Treatment of croup

Accurate diagnosis, gentle handling, and careful observation are the mainstays of good management. Children with croup are often frightened, miserable, and uncomfortable. Crying increases their oxygen demand and may increase laryngeal swelling. Gentle confident handling reassures the child and parents. Children are often happier on their parent's lap than lying flat on a cot. Disturbance of the child should be kept to a minimum.

Most cases of viral croup resolve spontaneously within 2–4 days. In others, increasing dyspnoea necessitates hospital admission.

Oxygen   Many children admitted to hospital with croup have hypoxaemia. The degree of hypoxaemia correlates poorly with clinical signs: the respiratory rate and the degree of sternal recession are the best indicators. Humidified oxygen should be given through a face-mask, and, if possible, the oxygen saturation monitored. Inhalation of warm moist air is widely used but is of unproven benefit.

Nebulised adrenaline   The role of nebulised adrenaline in severe croup remains controversial. Nebulised adrenaline (5 ml of 1:1000) given with oxygen through a face-mask will produce a transient improvement for 30–60 minutes, but rarely alters the long-term course of the illness. This treatment should only be given to children with signs of severe obstruction. Such children need to be observed very closely with continuous ECG and oxygen saturation monitoring, preferably on a paediatric intensive care unit, as they are likely to require endotracheal intubation. A marked tachycardia is usually produced, but other side effects are uncommon. This treatment is best used to "buy time" in which to assemble an experienced team to treat a child with severe croup.

Corticosteroids   There is no convincing evidence that systemic steroids produce a substantial benefit in the majority of children with croup, but they may be helpful in children with severe obstruction who require intubation (see below).

Endotracheal intubation   Up to 5% of children admitted to hospital with croup require endotracheal intubation. The decision to intubate is a clinical one based on increasing tachycardia, tachypnoea, and chest retraction, or the appearance of cyanosis, exhaustion, or confusion. Ideally, the procedure should be performed under general anaesthetic by an experienced paediatric anaesthetist, unless there has been a respiratory arrest. A much smaller gauge endotracheal tube than usual is often required. If there is doubt about the diagnosis, or difficulty in intubation is anticipated, an ENT surgeon capable of performing a tracheotomy should be present. Children with an endotracheal tube need meticulous care if complications such as tube blockage or displacement are to be avoided. The median duration of intubation in croup is 5 days: the younger the child, the longer the intubation usually required. Prednisolone (1 mg/kg every 12 hours) reduces the duration of intubation and the need for re-intubation in children with severe croup.

Acute epiglottitis

Acute epiglottitis shares many clinical features with croup but it should be regarded as a quite distinct entity. Although much less common than croup, its importance is that, unless the diagnosis is made rapidly and appropriate treatment commenced, total obstruction and death are likely to ensue.

Infection with *Haemophilus influenzae B* causes intense swelling of the epiglottis and the surrounding tissues, and obstruction of the larynx. Epiglottitis is most common in children aged 1–6 years, but it can occur in infants and in adults.

The onset of the illness is usually acute with high fever, lethargy, a soft inspiratory stridor, and rapidly increasing respiratory difficulty over 3–6 hours. In contrast to croup, cough is minimal or absent. Typically the child sits immobile, with his or her chin slightly raised and mouth open, drooling saliva. Such children look very toxic, pale and have poor peripheral circulation (most are septicaemic). There is usually a high fever (> 39°C). Because the throat is so painful, the child is reluctant to speak and unable to swallow drinks or saliva. Disturbance of the child, and particularly attempts to lie the child down to examine the throat with a spatula, or to insert an intravenous cannula, can precipitate total obstruction and death, and must be avoided.

The diagnosis of acute epiglottitis is made from the characteristic history and clinical findings. Lateral radiographs of the neck have been used to confirm the diagnosis, but these should be avoided as they disturb the child and have precipitated fatal total airway obstruction. Once the diagnosis is made, urgent admission to a paediatric intensive care unit should be arranged. The child will need intubation after careful gaseous induction of anaesthesia. When deeply anaesthetised the child can be laid on his or her back to allow laryngoscopy and intubation. Endotracheal intubation may be difficult because of the intense swelling and inflammation of the epiglottis ("cherry-red epiglottis"). Once the airway has been secured, blood should be sent for culture and treatment with intravenous chloramphenicol (25 mg/kg 6-hourly) or cefuroxime (30 mg/kg 8-hourly) commenced. With appropriate treatment, most children can be extubated after 24–36 hours and have recovered fully within 3–5 days. Complications such as hypoxic cerebral damage, pulmonary oedema, and other serious haemophilus infections are rare.

Table 8.2. Comparison of the clinical features of croup and epiglottitis

Feature	Croup	Epiglottitis
Onset	Over days	Over hours
Preceding coryza	Yes	No
Cough	Severe, barking	Absent or slight
Able to drink	Yes	No
Drooling saliva	No	Yes
Appearance	Unwell	Toxic, very ill
Fever	<38·5°C	>38·5°C
Stridor	Harsh, rasping	Soft
Voice	Hoarse	Reluctant to speak, muffled

Other causes of upper airway obstruction

Although croup and epiglottitis account for over 98% of cases of acute upper airway obstruction, several other uncommon conditions need to be considered in the differential diagnosis. *Diphtheria* is seen only in children who have not been immunised against the disease. Always ask about immunisations in any children with fever and the signs of upper airway obstruction, particularly if they have been abroad recently. Marked tonsillar swelling in *infectious mononucleosis* or *acute tonsillitis* can rarely compromise the upper airway. *Retropharyngeal abscess* is uncommon nowadays, but can present with fever and the features of upper airway obstruction. Surgical drainage and intravenous antibiotics are the treatment. Laryngeal oedema can develop over minutes as part of an *anaphylactic reaction*, often with angioneurotic oedema of the face and mouth. Food allergies, drug reactions, and insect stings are common causes of this. Oxygen, intravenous adrenaline, intravenous hydrocortisone, and an antihistamine are appropriate treatment, but intubation may be required.

The inquisitive and fearless toddler is at risk of inhaling a *foreign body*. Small toys, batteries, coins, and foodstuffs (nuts, sweets, meat) are the most common offending items. The object may pass through the larynx into the bronchial tree, where it produces a persistent cough of very acute onset, and unilateral wheezing. Examination of the chest may reveal decreased air entry on one side or evidence of a collapsed lung. Inspiratory and expiratory chest radiographs may show mediastinal shift on expiration due to gas trapping distal to the bronchial foreign body. Removal through a bronchoscope under general anaesthetic should be performed as soon as possible, because there is a risk of a cough moving the object into the trachea and causing more severe obstruction.

If an inhaled foreign body lodges in the larynx or trachea, the outcome is often fatal, unless measures, such as those discussed in Chapter 4, are performed. Should a child present with stridor and other signs of acute upper airway obstruction, and particularly if there is no fever or preceding illness, then a laryngeal foreign body is the probable diagnosis. Urgent removal of the object with a laryngoscope and Magill's forceps in the accident and emergency department may be life-saving.

LOWER AIRWAY OBSTRUCTION

Asthma

Acute exacerbation of asthma is the most common reason for a child to be admitted to hospital in this country. Admissions for acute asthma in children aged 0–4 years increased sevenfold between 1970 and 1986, and admissions for children in the 5–14 year age group tripled. Asthma now represents 10–20% of all acute medical admissions in children. There are 40–50 deaths from asthma in children each year. Consultations with general practitioners for symptoms of asthma have doubled in the last decade. These increases reflect a real increase in the prevalence of asthma in children.

History

The classic features of acute asthma are cough, wheeze, and breathlessness. An increase in these symptoms, and difficulty in walking, talking, or sleeping, all indicate worsening asthma. Decreasing relief from increasing doses of a bronchodilator always indicates worsening asthma.

Upper respiratory tract infections are the most common precipitant of symptoms of asthma in the pre-school child. Ninety per cent of these infections are caused by viruses. *Exercise*-induced symptoms are more frequent in the older child. Heat and water loss from the respiratory mucosa appears to be the mechanism by which exercise induces bronchoconstriction. Acute exacerbations may also be precipitated by *emotional upset, laughing*, or *excitement*. It is hard to assess the importance of *allergen exposure* to the onset of acute symptoms in an individual asthmatic child, partly because of the ubiquitous nature of the common allergens (house dust mite, grass pollens, moulds), and partly because delay in the allergic response makes a cause-and-effect relationship difficult to recognise. A rapid fall in *air temperature, exposure to a smoky atmosphere* and other *chemical irritants* such as paints, and domestic aerosols may trigger an acute attack.

Management of acute asthma

Assessment of severity   Except in the young infant, there is rarely any problem in making a diagnosis of acute asthma. An inhaled foreign body, bronchiolitis, croup, and acute epiglottitis should be considered as alternative diagnoses. It is difficult to assess the severity of an acute exacerbation. Important points in the history include the duration of symptoms, what treatment has already been given in this episode, and the course of previous attacks. Physical signs such as wheeze and respiratory rate are poor indicators of severity. Contraction of the sternomastoids, chest retraction, pulse rate, and the degree of pulsus paradoxus are better guides. Pulsus paradoxus (the difference between systolic pressure on inspiration and expiration) correlates well with measurements of airway obstruction: patients with more than 2·7 kPa (20 mmHg) of paradox have severe obstruction and require admission. Cyanosis is a late sign indicating life-threatening asthma.

The peak expiratory flow rate (PEFR) is a reliable measure of severity and should be a routine part of the assessment. Children below the age of 5 years, and those who are very dyspnoeic, are usually unable to produce reliable readings. Arterial oxygen saturation (Sao_2) is useful in assessing severity and predicting outcome in acute asthma. All children with a PEFR < 33% of their predicted value, or those with a saturation of less than 85%, require urgent treatment (see box). Other indications include a poor response to repeated doses of bronchodilator at home, or increasing exhaustion. A chest radiograph is indicated only if there is severe dyspnoea, uncertainty about the diagnosis, asymmetry of chest signs, or signs of severe infection. Measurement of arterial blood gases is indicated in severe or refractory cases.

Features of severe asthma

- Unable to talk in sentences
- Recession
- Peak flow <50% expected

Features of life-threatening asthma

- Conscious level depressed
- Severe recession
- Marked use of accessory muscles
- Oxygen saturation <85% in air
- Peak flow <33% expected
- Silent chest
- Cyanosis

Table 8.3.   Predicted values of peak expiratory flow rate in children

Height (cm)	Peak flow (l/min)
110	150
120	200
130	250
140	300
150	350
160	400
170	450

Treatment of acute asthma Nebulised β₂-bronchodilators, steroids, and oxygen form the foundation of the therapy of acute asthma. As soon as the diagnosis has been made, the child should be given nebulised *β₂-bronchodilator*. The nebuliser should be driven by oxygen (4–6 l/min) in all but the mildest of cases. This can be repeated every 1–2 hours until there is improvement. If nebulised treatment is unavailable, 10–20 puffs of a bronchodilator from a metered dose inhaler can be given through a spacer.

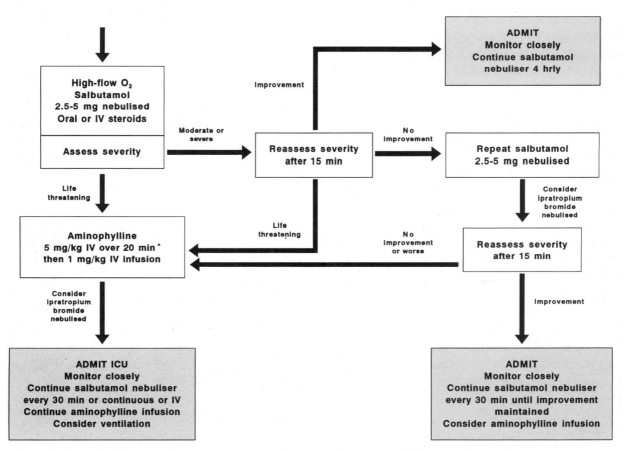

Figure 8.1. Algorithm for the management of acute asthma. *Omit if on oral theophylline

Corticosteroids expedite recovery from acute asthma. Although an oral single dose of prednisolone is effective, many paediatricians use a 3- to 5-day course. There is no need to taper off the dose, unless the child is on maintenance treatment with oral or high-dose inhaled steroids. Unless the child is vomiting, there is no advantage in giving steroids parenterally.

The increased use of nebulised bronchodilators and oral steroids has been associated with a reduction in the use of *intravenous aminophylline*. It still has a role in the child who fails to respond adequately to nebulised therapy. A loading dose is given over 15 minutes, followed by a continuous infusion. The pulse should be regularly checked for irregularities with continuous ECG monitoring during infusion of the loading dose. If the child has received slow-release theophylline in the previous 12 hours, the loading dose should be omitted. Seizures, severe vomiting, and fatal cardiac arrhythmias may follow rapid infusion. There is no place for rectal administration of these drugs, as absorption is unpredictable. *Intravenous fluids* should normally be restricted to approximately two-thirds of the normal daily requirements, as there is increased secretion of antidiuretic hormone in severe asthma. Antibiotics should only be given if there are clear signs of infection.

If the child fails to respond to the above measures, he or she should be moved to an *intensive care unit* as he or she will require continuous observation, and ECG and oxygen saturation monitoring. The frequency of nebulised β_2-bronchodilator should be increased to half-hourly, or, if necessary, be administered continuously. Although *intravenous salbutamol* normally offers no advantage over nebulised delivery, it has a place in life-threatening episodes that do not respond to nebulised therapy. Important side effects include sinus tachycardia and hypokalaemia: serum potassium levels should be checked 12-hourly. There is no convincing evidence that adding nebulised *ipratropium* (Atrovent) to maximal doses of β_2-bronchodilators is beneficial in severe acute asthma in children. It may be worth a trial if there is a poor response to nebulised β_2-bronchodilator, particularly in the infant.

Mechanical ventilation is rarely required. There are no absolute criteria for ventilation, but it should be considered if there is a carbon dioxide tension (P_{CO_2}) of >8 kPa, persistent hypoxaemia ($P_{O_2} <8$ kPa in an inspired oxygen of 60%), or increasing exhaustion, despite intensive drug therapy. In skilled hands, the prognosis is good but complications such as air leak and lobar collapse are common. Children with acute asthma who require mechanical ventilation should be transferred to a paediatric intensive care unit.

Table 8.4. Drugs used in treatment of acute asthma

Oxygen	High flow
Nebulised β_2-bronchodilator	Salbutamol 2·5–10 mg 1–4 hourly
	Terbutaline 5–10 mg 1–4 hourly
Prednisolone	2 mg/kg/day in two doses, for 3–5 days
	OR
	Intravenous hydrocortisone succinate
	loading dose 4 mg/kg
	continuous infusion 1 mg/kg/hour
Aminophylline	Loading dose 5 mg/kg intravenous over 15 minutes*
	Continuous infusion 1 mg/kg/h
Intravenous salbutamol	Loading dose 4–6 µg/kg over 10 min
	Continuous infusion 0·5–1·0 µg/kg/min
Nebulised ipratropium	125–250 µg 6-hourly

* Omit if child has received oral theophylline in previous 12 hours.

Whatever treatment is needed, it is important to monitor the response to treatment carefully. Assessment is based on physical signs and peak flow readings performed immediately before and 15–30 minutes after nebulised treatment. Oxygen saturation measurements offer a non-invasive, continuous, objective measurement of response. When there has been considerable improvement, intravenous treatment can be discontinued and the frequency of nebulised therapy reduced. The child's maintenance treatment should be reviewed and altered if inadequate. Inhaler technique should be checked.

BRONCHIOLITIS

Bronchiolitis is the most common, serious, respiratory infection of childhood: 2–3% of all infants are admitted to hospital with the disease each year. Ninety per cent of patients are aged 1–9 months: it is rare after 1 year of age. There is an annual winter epidemic. Respiratory syncytial virus is the pathogen in 75% of cases, the remainder of cases being caused by other respiratory viruses, such as parainfluenza, influenza, and adenoviruses. Acute bronchiolitis is never a primary bacterial infection, and it is likely that secondary bacterial involvement is rare.

Fever and a clear nasal discharge precede a dry cough and increasing breathlessness. Wheezing is often, but not always, present. Feeding difficulties associated with increasing dyspnoea are often the reason for admission to hospital. Recurrent apnoea is a serious and potentially fatal complication, and is seen particularly in infants born prematurely. Children with pre-existing chronic lung disease (e.g. cystic fibrosis, bronchopulmonary dysplasia in pre-term infants), and children with congenital heart disease are at particularly high risk of developing severe respiratory failure with bronchiolitis.

The findings on examination are characteristic.

Table 8.5. Bronchiolitis – characteristic findings on examination

Tachypnoea	50–100 breaths/minute
Recession	Subcostal and intercostal
Cough	Sharp, dry
Hyperinflation of the chest	Sternum prominent, liver depressed
Tachycardia	140–200 beats/minute
Crackles	Fine end-inspiratory
Wheezes	High-pitched expiratory > inspiratory
Colour	Cyanosis or pallor
Breathing pattern	Irregular breathing/recurrent apnoea

The chest radiograph shows hyperinflation with downward displacement and flattening of the diaphragm due to small airway obstruction and gas trapping. In one-third of infants there is also evidence of collapse or consolidation, particularly in the upper lobes. Respiratory syncytial virus can be cultured or identified with a fluorescent antibody technique on nasopharyngeal secretions. Blood gas analysis, which is required in only the most severe cases, shows lowered oxygen and raised carbon dioxide levels.

As there is no specific treatment for bronchiolitis, management is supportive. Humidified oxygen (30–50%) is delivered into a headbox, and intravenous or nasogastric fluids are commenced if required. Pulse oximetry is helpful in assessing the severity of hypoxaemia. Because of the risk of apnoea, small infants, and those with severe disease should be attached to oxygen saturation monitors. Antibiotics, bronchodilators, and steroids are of no value. The precise role of the nebulised antiviral agent ribavirin is unclear and its use should be reserved for children with pre-existing lung disease, those with impaired immunity, and infants with congenital heart disease. Mechanical ventilation is required in 2% of infants admitted to hospital, either because of recurrent apnoea, exhaustion, or hypercapnia and hypoxaemia secondary to severe small airway obstruction.

Most children recover from the acute infection within 2 weeks. However, as many as half will have recurrent episodes of cough and wheeze over the next 3–5 years. Rarely, there is severe permanent damage to the airways (bronchiolitis obliterans).

PNEUMONIA

Pneumonia in childhood is still responsible for over 150 deaths each year. Infants, and children with congenital abnormalities or chronic illnesses, are at particular risk. In adults, two-thirds of cases of pneumonia are caused by either pneumococci or *Haemophilus influenzae*. A much wider spectrum of pathogens causes pneumonia in childhood, and different organisms are important in different age groups.

In the *newborn*, organisms from the mother's genital tract, such as *Eschericia coli* and other Gram-negative bacilli, group B β-haemolytic streptococci and, increasingly, *Chlamydia trachomatis*, are the most common pathogens. In *infancy* respiratory viruses, particularly respiratory syncytial virus, are the most frequent cause, but pneumococci, *Haemophilus* sp., and, less commonly, *Staphylococcus aureus* are also important. In *older children*, viruses become less frequent pathogens and bacterial infection is more important. *Mycoplasma pneumoniae* is a common cause of pneumonia in the school-age child.

Diagnosis

Fever, cough, breathlessness, and lethargy following an upper respiratory infection are the usual presenting symptoms. The cough is often dry initially but then becomes loose. Older children may produce purulent sputum, but in those below the age of 5 years it is usually swallowed. Pleuritic chest pain, neck stiffness, and abdominal pain may be present if there is pleural inflammation. Classic signs of consolidation such as impaired percussion, decreased breath sounds, and bronchial breathing are often absent, particularly in infants, and a chest radiograph is needed. This may show lobar consolidation, widespread bronchopneumonia, or, less commonly, cavitation of the lung. Pleural effusions are quite common, particularly in bacterial pneumonia. Blood cultures, swabs for viral isolation, and a full blood count should also be performed.

Treatment

As it is not possible to differentiate reliably between bacterial or viral infection on clinical or radiological grounds, all children diagnosed as having pneumonia should receive antibiotics (Table 8.6). The initial choice of antibiotics depends on the age of the child. Antibiotics should be given for 7–10 days, except in staphylococcal pneumonia, where a course of 4–6 weeks' duration is needed. Many older children have no respiratory difficulty and can be treated at home. Infants, and children who look toxic or have definite dyspnoea, should be admitted. Physiotherapy, an adequate fluid intake, and oxygen (in severe pneumonia) are also required. Mechanical ventilation is rarely required unless there is a serious underlying condition. If a child has recurrent or persistent pneumonia, investigations to exclude underlying conditions such as cystic fibrosis or immunodeficiency should be performed.

Table 8.6. Drug treatment for pneumonia

Age	Most common bacterial pathogens	Antibiotics
Newborn (<4 weeks)	Suspected bacterial infection	Intravenous benzylpenicillin+gentamicin or Intravenous cefotaxime
	Suspected chlamydial infection	Intravenous erythromycin
Infants and toddlers	Pneumococci	Intravenous benzylpenicillin
	Haemophilus sp.	Intravenous amoxycillin
	Staphylococcus aureus	Intravenous flucloxacillin
Age 2–12 years	Pneumococci	Intravenous benzylpenicillin
	Haemophilus sp.	Intravenous or oral amoxycillin
	Mycoplasma sp.	Intravenous or oral erythromycin

CONCLUSIONS

Despite recent advances in diagnosis and management, respiratory illness remains an important cause of morbidity and death in childhood. Many of the deaths are potentially avoidable with prompt and accurate diagnosis, and optimal treatment. Reliable assessment of the cause and severity of respiratory emergencies depends on meticulous clinical examination and a clear understanding of the underlying pathology.

9

Shock

DEFINITION

Shock results from an acute failure of circulatory function. Inadequate amounts of nutrients, especially oxygen, are delivered to body tissues and there is inadequate removal of tissue waste products. Shock is a complex clinical syndrome that is the body's response to cellular metabolic deficiency.

The initial haemodynamic abnormality of fluid loss or fluid shift is followed by compensatory mechanisms under neuroendocrine control. Later, shock is worsened by the production of vasoactive mediators and the products of cellular breakdown. The identity and relative importance of these chemicals are as yet poorly understood.

THE THREE PHASES OF SHOCK

Compensated
uncompensated
Irreversible

Shock is a progressive syndrome but it can be divided into three phases: compensated, uncompensated, and irreversible. Although artificial, this division is useful because each phase has characteristic clinicopathological manifestations and outcome.

Phase 1: (compensated) shock

In this phase vital organ function (brain and heart) is conserved by sympathetic reflexes which increase systemic arterial resistance, divert blood away from non-essential tissues, constrict the venous reservoir, and increase the heart rate to maintain cardiac output. The systolic blood pressure remains normal whereas the diastolic pressure may be elevated due to increased systemic arterial resistance. Increased secretion of angiotensin and vasopressin allows the kidneys to conserve water and salt, and intestinal fluid is reabsorbed from the digestive tract. Clinical signs at this stage include mild agitation or confusion, skin pallor, increased heart rate, and cold peripheral skin with decreased capillary return.

Phase 2: (uncompensated) shock

In uncompensated shock, the compensatory mechanisms start to fail and the circulatory system is no longer efficient. Areas that have poor perfusion can no longer metabolise aerobically, and anaerobic metabolism becomes their major source of energy production. Anaerobic metabolism is comparatively inefficient. Only 2 moles adenosine triphosphate (ATP) are produced for each mole of glucose metabolised compared to 38 moles of ATP per mole of glucose metabolised aerobically.

Anaerobic pathways produce excess lactate leading to systemic acidosis. The acidosis is compounded by intracellular carbonic acid formed because of the inability of the circulation to remove CO_2. Acidosis reduces myocardial contractility and impairs the response to catecholamines.

A further result of anaerobic metabolism is the failure of the energy-dependent sodium–potassium pump, which maintains the normal homoeostatic environment in which the cell functions.

Lysosomal, mitochondrial, and membrane functions deteriorate without this homoeostasis. Sluggish flow of blood and chemical changes in small vessels lead to platelet adhesion, and may produce damaging chain reactions in the kinin and coagulation systems leading to a bleeding tendency.

Mediators

Numerous chemical mediators have been identified in shocked patients, but the roles of each have not been clearly identified. They include histamine, serotonin, cytokines (especially tumour necrosis factor and interleukin 1), xanthine oxidase (which generates oxygen radicals), platelet-aggregating factor, and bacterial toxins. They are largely produced by cells of the immune system, especially monocytic macrophages. It has been suggested that these mediators, which developed as initial adaptive responses to severe injury and illness, may have deleterious consequences in the "unnatural" setting of the resuscitated patient. When the role of these chemical mediators is more fully understood, blocking agents may be produced which will improve the treatment in phase 2 shock.

The result of these cascading metabolic changes is to reduce tissue perfusion and oxidation further. Blood pools in some areas because arterioles can no longer control flow in the capillary system. Furthermore, abnormal capillary permeability allows further fluid loss from the circulation into the interstitium.

Clinically, the patient in phase 2 shock has a falling blood pressure, very slow capillary return, tachycardia, cold peripheries, acidotic breathing, depressed cerebral state, and absent urine output.

Phase 3: (irreversible) shock

The diagnosis of irreversible shock is a retrospective one. The damage to key organs such as the heart and brain is of such magnitude that death occurs despite adequate restoration of the circulation. Pathophysiologically, the high-energy phosphate reserves in cells (especially those of the liver and heart) are greatly diminished. The ATP has been degraded via adenosine to uric acid. New ATP is synthesised at only 2% an hour and the body can be said to have run out of energy. This underlies the clinical observation that during the progression of shock a point is reached at which death of the patient is inevitable, despite therapeutic intervention. *Hence early recognition and effective treatment of shock are vital.*

CAUSES OF SHOCK

Maintenance of adequate tissue perfusion depends on a pump (the heart) delivering the correct type and volume of fluid (blood) through controlled vessels (arteries, veins, and capillaries) without abnormal obstruction to flow. Inadequate tissue perfusion

74

resulting in impaired cellular respiration (i.e. shock) may result from defects of the pump (cardiogenic), loss of fluid (hypovolaemic), abnormalities of vessels (distributive), flow restriction (obstructive), or inadequate oxygen-releasing capacity (dissociative).

From the box it can be seen that the most common causes of shock in the paediatric patient are hypovolaemia from any cause, septicaemia, and the effects of trauma.

Classification of causes of shock (common causes are emboldened)

Hypovolaemic
Haemorrhage
Diarrhoea
Vomiting
Burns
Peritonitis
Distributive
Septicaemia
Anaphylaxis
Vasodilating drugs
Anaesthesia
Spinal cord injury
Cardiogenic
Arrhythmias
Cardiomyopathy
Heart failure
Valvular disease
Myocardial contusion
Myocardial infarction
Obstructive
Tension pneumothorax
Haemopneumothorax
Flail chest
Cardiac tamponade
Pulmonary embolism
Hypertension
Dissociative
Profound anaemia
Carbon monoxide poisoning
Methaemoglobinaemia

CLINICAL MANIFESTATIONS OF SHOCK

History

The history is vital in treating the shocked patient. Knowledge of the child's previous illnesses and the history of the present illness or injury will give important clues as to the underlying cause of the shocked state – necessary in order to direct therapy appropriately.

Examination

The physical signs of shock
Heart rate   A raised heart rate is a common response to many types of stress (fever, anxiety, hypoxia, hypovolaemia). In shock, tachycardia is caused by catecholamine release, and is an attempt to maintain cardiac output by increasing heart rate in the face

of falling stroke volume. *Bradycardia in a shocked child is caused by hypoxia and acidosis and is a pre-terminal sign.*

Hypotension Children's cardiovascular systems compensate well initially in shock. *Hypotension is a late and often sudden sign of decompensation and, if not reversed, will be rapidly followed by death.*

Especially in young infants blood pressure is a difficult measure to obtain and interpret. A formula for calculating systolic blood pressure is:

$$80 + (2 \times \text{Age in years})$$

Serial measurements of blood pressure should be performed frequently and any observed fall treated vigorously.

Peripheral pulses Examination of the peripheral circulation can give early warning of imminent decompensation. Diminished peripheral pulse volume suggests reduced stroke volume. In early septic shock there is sometimes a high output state which will produce bounding pulses.

Skin perfusion Poor skin perfusion is a useful early sign of shock. Slow capillary refill (>2 seconds) after blanching pressure for 5 seconds is evidence of reduced skin perfusion. When testing for capillary refill, the extremity should be lifted slightly above the level of the heart. Mottling, pallor, and peripheral cyanosis also indicate poor skin perfusion. All these signs may be difficult to interpret in patients who have just been exposed to cold.

A core/toe temperature difference of more than 2°C is a sign of poor skin perfusion.

Ventilation The acidosis produced by poor tissue perfusion in shock leads to rapid deep breathing.

Mental status Early signs of brain hypoperfusion are agitation and confusion, often alternating with drowsiness. Infants may be irritable but drowsy with a weak cry and hypotonia. They may not focus on the parent's face. These are important early cerebral signs of shock. Later the child becomes progressively drowsier until consciousness is lost.

Urine output Urine flow is decreased or absent in shock. It is not a useful initial assessment but hourly measurement is helpful in monitoring progress. A minimum flow of 1 ml/kg/h in children and 2 ml/kg/h in infants indicates adequate renal perfusion.

Rapid circulatory assessment

Heart rate
Blood pressure
Peripheral pulses
   Absent/present
   Volume
Skin perfusion
   Capillary refill time
   Peripheral skin temperature
   Colour
   Mottling – absent/present
Mental status
   Recognise parents
   Reaction to pain
   Muscle tone

Frequent re-evaluation of signs is vital to detect deterioration or improvement.

GENERAL MANAGEMENT OF SHOCK

1. Maintain a patent, protected airway.
2. Ventilation (spontaneous or supported) should be given with oxygen at a concentration of as near 100% as possible.
3. Obtain venous or intraosseous access.
4. Give crystalloid 20 ml/kg immediately.
5. Take blood for haematocrit, urea and electrolytes, culture, cross-match, glucose.
6. Improve circulatory status by:
    (a) optimising preload: in hypovolaemic shock, the most common cause of shock in the paediatric age group, circulating volume, should be increased.
    (b) improving cardiac contractility: for a discussion of drugs affecting the heart see Chapter 10;
    (c) decreasing afterload: this involves reducing the resistance to blood flow from the heart or relieving a physical obstruction such as a pneumothorax or cardiac tamponade following trauma (see Chapter 15);
    (d) improving oxygen-carrying capacity, especially in cases when there has been blood loss, shock may not be reversed until the oxygen-carrying capacity has been increased by blood transfusion, even though fluid volume is restored.

SEQUELAE OF SHOCK

During and following successful restoration of circulation, varying degrees of organ damage may remain, and should be actively sought and managed.

Kidneys

Prerenal failure, acute tubular necrosis, and the more severe cortical necrosis may be sequelae of phase 2 shock. Once haemodynamic parameters are improving, fluid administration should be reviewed and serum electrolytes, urea, and creatinine analysed.

Lung

"Shock lung" (adult respiratory distress syndrome) appears to be a more common sequel in adults than in children. Patients with this complication develop respiratory failure because of increased lung water caused by hydrostatic oedema and permeability oedema. Ventilation with high inspired oxygen is necessary, and positive end-expiratory pressure (PEEP) may be required.

Heart

Despite adequate volume restoration, and even if shock was not primarily cardiogenic, poor myocardial perfusion often leads to decreased contractility. Inotropic agents and intensive monitoring may then be required (see Chapter 10).

Coagulation abnormalities

As described above, sludging of blood and the production of chemical mediators may initiate microvascular clotting which leads to a consumption coagulopathy. Clotting times and a platelet count should be estimated and fresh frozen plasma given if clinically indicated.

Other organs

The liver and bowel may be damaged in shock, leading to gastrointestinal bleeding. Endocrine organs may be variously affected and patients must be monitored for glucose and mineral homoeostasis. However, it is probably the extent of irreversible brain damage that is most anxiously monitored by the carers of a shocked patient, because the brain is the most sensitive of all organs to hypoxia and ischaemia.

SPECIFIC SHOCK SYNDROMES

Hypovolaemic shock

Hypovolaemia is the most common cause of shock in infancy and childhood, and results from loss of circulating volume from any cause. Specific causes are summarised in the box. The keys to successful resuscitation are *early recognition* and *aggressive fluid replacement*.

Examples of causes of hypovolaemic shock

Blood loss
    External haemorrhage, e.g. lacerations/open fractures
    Internal haemorrhage, e.g. ruptured spleen/closed fractures
Loss of plasma
    Burns
Dehydration
    Gastroenteritis
    Peritonitis
    Diabetes mellitus/insipidus
    Ileostomy losses

Normal values
Vital signs   The normal values for vital signs are summarised in Table 9.1.

Table 9.1. Vital signs: approximate range of normal

Age (years)	Respiratory rate (breaths/min)	Systolic BP (mmHg)	Pulse (/min)
<1	30–40	70–90	110–160
2–5	25–30	80–100	95–140
5–12	20–25	90–110	80–120
>12	15–20	100–120	60–100

All single parameters should be interpreted within the whole clinical context.

Weight and blood volume   These can be calculated using the following formulae:

$$\text{Weight in kg} = 2\,(\text{Age in years} + 4)$$
$$\text{Blood volume (ml)} = 80 \times \text{weight in kg}$$

Clinical signs of hypovolaemic shock Data on the stages of shock in infants and children are limited, but the clinical signs shown in Table 9.2 are useful in the assessment of hypovolaemic shock.

Table 9.2. Signs of shock from blood loss

	Compensated	Uncompensated	Pre-terminal (?irreversible)
Blood loss (%)	Up to 25	25–40	>40
Heart rate	Tachycardia+	Tachycardia++	Tachycardia/bradycardia
Systolic BP	Normal	Normal or falling	Plummeting
Pulse volume	Normal/reduced	Reduced+	Reduced++
Capillary refill time (Normal <2 s)	Normal/increased	Increased+	Increased++
Skin	Cool, pale	Cold, mottled	Cold, deathly pale
Respiratory rate	Tachypnoea+	Tachypnoea++	Sighing respiration
Mental state	Mild agitation	Lethargic Uncooperative	Reacts only to pain or unresponsive

Circulatory access

A short, wide-bore peripheral venous or intraosseous cannula should be used. Upper central venous lines are unsuitable for the resuscitation of hypovolaemic children because of the risk of iatrogenic pneumothorax, or exacerbation of an unsuspected neck injury; both these complications can be fatal. Femoral vein access is safer, if peripheral or intraosseous access is impossible.

Take blood for haemoglobin, haematocrit, blood sugar, urea and electrolytes, and cross-match.

Routes for vascular access are described in Chapter 22.

Fluid volume and type
- An initial fluid bolus of 20 ml/kg is given as fast as possible.
- This should be repeated after assessment if there is no improvement in vital signs.
- The most common mistake in the treatment of hypovolaemic shocked children is failure to give enough fluid.

Crystalloid or colloid fluids are available for volume replacement. Colloids diffuse less readily into the interstitial space and therefore more effectively expand the intravascular volume with the use of smaller volumes. Proponents of the use of crystalloids suggest that the interstitial space is already depleted in hypovolaemia because of shifts of fluids from the interstitial space into the intravascular and intracellular compartments. It is also thought that, when colloids do leak into the interstitial space, their high osmotic pressure increases the fluid loss from capillaries into the interstitial space.

When crystalloids are used the volume required is two to three times that of a colloid. As crystalloids leak into the interstitial space, it is not uncommon for tissue oedema to occur. There is disagreement as to whether the oedema is detrimental to tissue oxygenation or not. Clearly the decision to use a particular type of fluid to replace volume loss needs to take into account the cause of hypovolaemia. Often, the use of both crystalloid and colloid is appropriate. Further details on the composition of fluids, their advantages and disadvantages can be found in Appendix B.

If blood is needed, it may be given after full cross-match which takes about 1 hour to perform. In more urgent situations type-specific non-cross-matched blood (which is

ABO rhesus compatible but has a higher incidence of transfusion reactions) should be requested. It takes about 15 minutes to prepare. In dire emergencies O-negative blood must be given.

Fluids should be *warmed* if time permits. Isotonic electrolyte solution should be kept available in a warmed cabinet. Further details on the management of shock in trauma burns and diabetes can be found in Chapters 19, 14, and Appendix B respectively.

Further management Intubation and ventilation should be strongly considered in a patient who has failed to respond adequately to two boluses of fluid (i.e. half the estimated intravascular volume).

Check *arterial blood gases* and consider correcting metabolic acidosis if the pH is less than 7·15 and is not improving after improved perfusion. These patients should be ventilated.

Surgery may be necessary as part of the emergency treatment of haemorrhagic shock from trauma, and, in such cases, early consultation is vital.

Monitoring

All the *vital signs* tabled above, particularly the capillary refill time, must be reassessed repeatedly to follow response to treatment.

Urine output should be maintained at over 2 ml/kg/h in infants and 1 ml/kg/h in older children.

Central venous pressure monitoring will help monitor fluid resuscitation in refractory cases, but bear in mind the risks of subclavian placement. The femoral vein is safer for the inexperienced (see Chapter 22).

Pitfalls in diagnosis

Hypovolaemic shock should never be attributed to an isolated head injury in a child, though an infant may have a subgaleal haematoma of sufficient volume to cause hypovolaemia. An infant with a patent fontanelle can lose a considerable volume of blood within the cranium as the cranium allows for expansion. In trauma, if hypovolaemia is unexplained, occult blood loss should be considered. This may be intraperitoneal, retroperitoneal, or intrathoracic.

Hypoglycaemia may give a similar clinical picture to that of compensated shock. This must always be excluded by urgent glucose stick test and blood glucose estimation. Hypoglycaemia and hypovolaemia may coexist.

Frequent careful monitoring of the child's vital signs with repeated reassessment and re-examination are mandatory.

Anaphylactic shock

Anaphylaxis is a potentially life-threatening syndrome which may progress to shock. It is immunologically mediated. The most common causes are allergy to penicillin, to radiographic contrast media, and to certain foods, especially nuts.

Prodromal symptoms of flushing, itching, facial swelling, urticaria, abdominal pain, diarrhoea, wheeze, and stridor may precede shock or may be the only manifestations of anaphylaxis.

Management of anaphylactic shock

Anaphylactic shock is caused by acute vasodilatation and by fluid loss from the intravascular space caused by increased capillary permeability. The immediate management centres on the administration of adrenaline and aggressive fluid resuscitation (Figure 9.1).

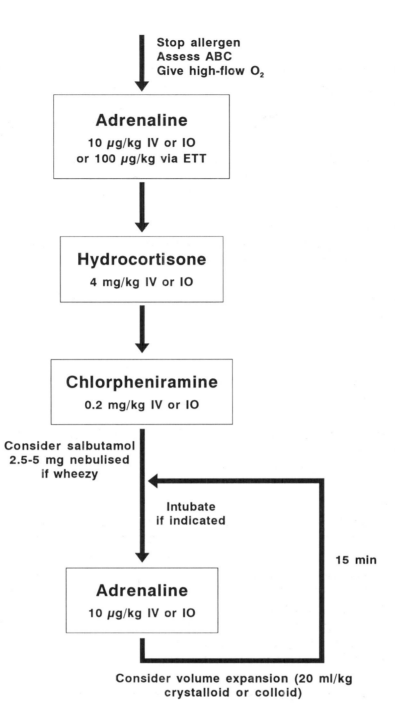

Figure 9.1. Protocol for the management of anaphylaxis

If boluses of adrenaline are not effective, give an infusion of adrenaline $0 \cdot 1$–$5 \cdot 0\ \mu g/kg/$ min. If bronchospasm is a feature give $2 \cdot 5$–10 mg nebulised salbutamol initially; continuously nebulised salbutamol can be used if required. Ventilation may be necessary.

Septic shock

In sepsis the cardiac output may be normal or raised, but may still be too small to deliver sufficient oxygen to the tissues. This is because abnormal distribution of blood in the microcirculation leads to decreased tissue perfusion.

Other causes of maldistribution in children include anaphylaxis, spinal cord injury, and drug intoxication (especially barbiturates). Sepsis is the most important cause, however, and is the source of considerable morbidity and mortality.

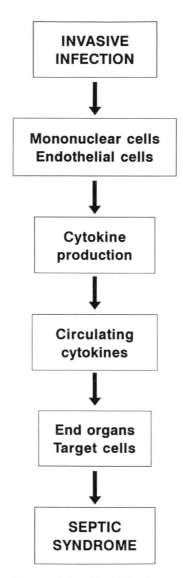

Figure 9.2. Simplified mechanism of septic shock

The release of bacterial toxins triggers complex interacting haemodynamic and metabolic changes. Mediators and activators are released and react to produce the "septic syndrome". These activators may be vasodilators or vasoconstrictors; some promote and activate the coagulation cascade; others are cardiac depressants.

In septic shock cardiac function may be depressed. Oxygen delivery to the heart from the coronary arteries occurs mainly in diastole, and the tachycardia and increased oxygen demand of the myocardium in septic shock may jeopardise cardiac oxygenation. Metabolic acidosis also damages myocardial cells at mitochondrial level. The function of the left ventricle is affected more than the right ventricle. This may be due to myocardial oedema, adrenogenic receptor dysfunction, or impaired sarcolemmal calcium influx. The right ventricle is less important in maintaining cardiac output than the left, but increased pulmonary vascular resistance can limit the hyperdynamic state and oxygen delivery.

In septic shock cells do not use oxygen properly. There appears to be a block at the mitochondrial level in the mechanism of oxygen uptake, and in progressive shock the difference between arterial and venous saturation levels of oxygen is inappropriately narrow. This progressive deterioration in cell oxygen consumption heralds multiple organ failure.

82

Early (compensated) septic shock

This is characterised by a raised cardiac output, decreased systemic resistance, warm extremities, and a wide pulse pressure. This hyperdynamic state is recognised by hyperpyrexia, hyperventilation, tachycardia, and mental confusion. All of these signs may be minimal: mental confusion in particular needs to be looked for carefully, if septic shock is not to be overlooked at this stage.

Late (uncompensated) septic shock

If no effective therapy is given, the cardiovascular performance deteriorates and cardiac output diminishes. Even with a normal or raised cardiac output, shock develops. The normal relationship between cardiac output and systemic vascular resistance breaks down and hypotension may persist as a result of decreased vascular resistance.

The cardiac output may fall gradually over several hours, or precipitously in minutes. As tissue hypoxia develops, plasma lactic acid levels increase.

Infants who have little cardiac reserve often present with hypotension and a hypodynamic picture. These sick babies are a diagnostic challenge but sepsis must be assumed and treated as quickly as possible.

Survival in septic shock depends on the maintenance of a hyperdynamic state. Several factors mitigate against this by encouraging hypovolaemia:

1. Increased microvascular permeability.
2. Arteriolar and venous dilatation with peripheral pooling of blood.
3. Inadequate fluid intake.
4. Fluid loss secondary to fever, diarrhoea, and vomiting.
5. Inappropriate polyuria.

Causes of septic shock

The main pathogens in septic shock are Gram-negative bacteria, but β-haemolytic streptococci, staphylococci, and other Gram-positive bacteria are also of importance. *Neisseria meningitides* and *Haemophilus influenzae* are the two most common bacterial causes of septic shock in previously well children.

Every effort must be made to find a focus of infection which could be the source of the illness. A careful examination includes a search for purpuric spots which make the presumptive diagnosis of meningococcaemia highly likely.

Differential diagnosis of a "septic looking" child Various medical problems can mimic the clinical signs of septic shock. These are summarised in the box.

Medical problem	Examples
Cardiac abnormalities	Dysrhythmias
	Myocarditis
	Cardiomyopathies
Congenital heart disease	
Metabolic disorders	Inborn errors of metabolism
	Hypoglycaemia or electrolyte disturbances
Gastrointestinal disturbances	Gastrointestinal obstruction or ischaemia, e.g. volvulus, intussusception
	Gastroenteritis with dehydration
Severe child abuse (the shaken child syndrome)	
Severe anaemia	Haemolytic uraemic syndrome
Reye's syndrome	
Haemorrhagic shock encephalopathy syndrome	

Treatment in septic shock

Oxygen   Give 100% oxygen by mask. Consider assisted ventilation if the patient's respiratory effort is great and tiring or appears to be inadequate despite oxygen therapy.

Fluids   Give a bolus of fluid (20 ml/kg) and repeat if there is no clinical improvement. Colloids are more successful in septic shock than crystalloids, as the latter leak quickly out of the vascular compartment. Over 60 ml/kg of colloid may be needed.

Antibiotics   It is customary to give penicillin and a third-generation cephalosporin such as cefotaxime until sensitivities are known. Other pathogens suspected because of a specific history must be treated appropriately and urgently.

In neonatal sepsis ampicillin and gentamicin or ampicillin and cefotaxime are given until therapy can be guided by the laboratory.

Other drugs

Inotropic agents   If perfusion is still poor after colloid 60 ml/kg has been given or if a central venous pressure reading shows a level of over 1·33 kPa (10 mmHg) then inotropes may be necessary. Adrenaline or isoprenaline, by infusion, are useful for poorly contracting myocardium or bradycardia. Isoprenaline increases cardiac oxygen requirements and its benefit must be weighed against this. Dopamine with or without dobutamine may improve cardiac output and protect renal function while not increasing cardiac work and oxygen requirement excessively. In late septic shock, in which there is increased cardiac filling pressure and a poor cardiac output, sodium nitroprusside, which causes a peripheral vasodilatation, may be of benefit (see Chapter 10).

Sodium bicarbonate   This may be necessary to counteract a metabolic acidosis but only if severe acidosis (pH < 7·15) persists after adequate fluid replacement. Bicarbonate therapy must be monitored biochemically and the patient must be ventilated.

Calcium   Decreased plasma concentrations of ionised calcium may occur in sepsis and should be corrected when identified. However, remember that calcium can cause bradycardia and local tissue damage.

Glucose   Hypoglycaemia must be sought and corrected with 25% glucose. This problem is very common in young septic infants as they often have had a low calorie intake and have poor glycogen stores.

Monitoring

State of consciousness – Glasgow Coma Scale
Respiratory rate
Core temperature
Cardiovascular parameters
  Skin and core temperature difference
  Pulse rate and volume
  Blood pressure
  Capillary perfusion time
  Central venous pressure – should be monitored in a patient where there has been poor
  response to fluid therapy or with established shock. Note that the central venous pressure
  does not necessarily reflect left ventricular filling pressure and may be misleading
Urinary output – urine bag, or preferably catheter; output should be 1–2 ml/kg body weight
Pulse oximetry

Investigations
Blood tests
- Blood glucose*.
- Full blood count and differential.
- Urea and electrolytes*, to include calcium and phosphate levels.
- Clotting screen.
- Blood culture.
- Blood gases and pH*.
- Group and save, in case blood transfusion becomes necessary.

Other tests which may be needed
- Lumbar puncture.
- Urine culture.
- Appropriate swabs.
- Chest radiograph.

* These tests need to be repeated frequently as the clinical picture dictates.

Key points in management

- Remember BP and pulse are unreliable indicators in early sepsis
- Look for minor degrees of mental impairment (anxiety, restlessness)
- Do not delay treatment, try to prevent the onset of hypotension, metabolic acidosis, and hypoxia
- Give adequate fluids early in treatment, especially colloids
- Do not use inotropic agents until the patient has received adequate fluid therapy
- Monitor blood glucose, gases, and pH, and treat appropriately

---

SOME SPECIFIC CONDITIONS

Meningococcal septicaemia

Meningococcal septicaemia is the most fulminant infectious disease. The interval from first symptom to death can be less than 12 hours. Some patients complain of a sore throat at the onset of the disease; others are simply febrile and ill. The cardinal sign of meningococcal septicaemia is a purpuric rash in an ill child. At the onset, the rash is not florid and a careful search should be made for purpura in any unwell child. In about 10% of patients with meningococcal septicaemia, an initial blanching erythematous rash precedes a purpuric one, and in some cases no rash occurs.

Purpura is caused by vasculitis and disseminated intravascular coagulation (DIC), the result of endotoxins produced by the organism *Neisseria meningitides*, and the presence of circulating cytokines. Although the majority of patients who survive have no long-term sequelae, a few have skin or limb loss as a result of vasculitis and DIC.

Management
If meningococcal septicaemia is suspected, a blood culture and full blood count should be taken, and intravenous benzylpenicillin 50 mg/kg (up to a maximum of 2 g) and a third-generation cephalosporin such as cefotaxime should be given immediately. The antibiotics should be administered over 5–10 minutes, as more rapid infusion of such a high dose of penicillin could cause convulsions. Treat shock as described.

85

Toxic shock syndrome

This condition is caused by a phage group 1 staphylococcal or occasionally a group A haemolytic streptococcal infection. It is uncommon, but can occur in burned and scalded patients or those with skin abrasions, whatever the size and depth of their injury. It can also occur in vaginal tampon users. The clinical picture includes a high fever, headache, confusion, conjunctival and mucosal hyperaemia, scarlatiniform rash with secondary desquamation, subcutaneous oedema, vomiting, watery diarrhoea, hepatic and renal damage, disseminated intravascular coagulation, and severe prolonged shock.

Patients with toxic shock syndrome require shock management and antibiotics, such as flucloxacillin or penicillin and a third-generation cephalosporin.

Haemorrhagic shock encephalopathy syndrome

This is a shock syndrome of unknown but non-infectious origin in young children. It is rare but has an extremely poor outcome with a mortality of about 50% and severe neurological damage in most survivors. There are some resemblances to the illness caused by overheating.

The presentation is abrupt and severe. Previously well or only mildly ill babies are discovered extremely ill in their cots. Symptoms include bloody diarrhoea, coma, convulsions, and shock.

Hepatomegaly and anuria or oliguria are usually found. Hypoglycaemia and a bleeding tendency are shown on blood testing.

Initial management of these babies is challenging. Treatment is required to control convulsions (Chapter 11), reverse shock (Chapter 9), and hypoglycaemia (Chapter 11) while reducing intracranial pressure (Chapter 17).

10

Cardiac emergencies

This chapter addresses the recognition and management of the following:

- Rhythm disturbances (excluding arrest rhythms which are discussed in Chapter 6).
- Cardiogenic shock.
- Duct-dependent congenital heart lesions.
- Acute pulmonary outflow tract obstruction.
- Systemic hypertension.
- Heart failure.

ARRHYTHMIA: RECOGNITION AND MANAGEMENT

Arrhythmia recognition

When a child presents in shock or in imminent cardiac failure due to a rhythm abnormality, it is not necessary to understand the subtleties of the presenting rhythm. Immediate management and medication will depend on a few simple criteria, as shown in the box.

> 1. Is the child stable or in shock?
> 2. Is the *rate*:
>   too fast?
>   too slow?
> 3. Is the *rhythm*:
>   regular?
>   irregular?
> 4. Are the *QRS complexes*:
>   narrow?
>   broad?

The diagnosis is made by cardiac monitor (lead II) or/and a 12-lead ECG. Check the rhythm on at least two leads.

Rate and regularity

Is the rate too fast?

Sinus tachycardia (Figure 10.1) can cause the heart rate to rise as high as 220/minute in an infant. It is often caused by fever or dehydration and a history may be obtained of recent illness. The rate may be *variable*; the rhythm is regular. Each QRS complex is preceded by a P wave. All P waves and QRS complexes are identical.

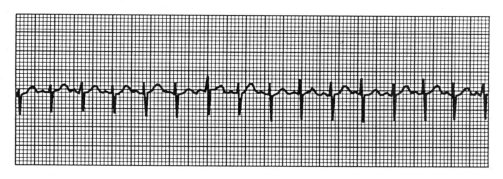

Figure 10.1. Sinus tachycardia

Supraventricular tachycardia (Figure 10.2) gives rise to a heart rate over 220/min, and often up to 300/min in an infant. The rhythm is *regular* and the QRS complexes are uniform in appearance. Each QRS is preceded by a P wave but these may not be visible due to the tachycardia.

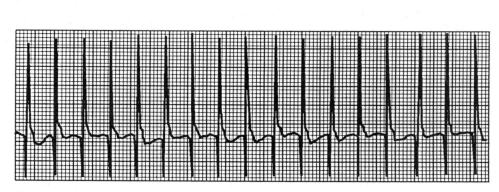

Figure 10.2. Supraventricular tachycardia

The onset and cessation of supraventricular tachycardia are sudden. The rhythm may last for only a few minutes or up to several days. It is tolerated remarkably well by some children, but an infant may present with poor feeding, sweating, poor colour, peripheral vasoconstriction, hepatomegaly, and other signs of cardiac failure. The supraventricular tachycardia may occasionally degenerate into ventricular fibrillation.

Supraventricular tachycardia is the most common primary cardiac arrhythmia in infancy and childhood. The majority of cases have a re-entry tachycardia with aberrant conduction through the atrioventricular node and an accessory pathway. When the tachycardia has been treated, and sinus rhythm is resumed, a Wolff–Parkinson–White phenomenon may be revealed on an ECG recording. This is a slow upstroke to the QRS, called a delta wave. Re-entry tachycardias without a delta wave but with a short P–R interval have the Lown–Ganong–Levine syndrome. Abnormal pathways can occur with Ebstein's anomaly, corrected transposition, or cardiomyopathies, but 70–80% of patients have a structurally normal heart.

In a few patients with supraventricular tachycardia the QRS complex is wide due to slow ventricular conduction. However, in most cases of wide complex tachycardia a ventricular focus is the cause.

Ventricular tachycardia (Figure 10.3) is defined as three or more ectopic ventricular beats and is termed "sustained" if it continues for longer than 30 seconds. The rate varies between 120 and 250 beats/min and the QRS complexes are *almost regular* though wide in appearance. As the beats originate in the ventricle and are not conducted down the bundle of His, the QRS complex is wide and there is no preceding P wave. It is an uncommon rhythm in children. When present there is usually an underlying cause. This may be primarily cardiac as in myocarditis, cardiomyopathy, or in a patient with congenital heart disease, especially after surgery. Other causes of ventricular tachycardia include poisoning with drugs that prolong the Q–T interval such as proteinamide and quinidine, and with psychotropic drugs such as phenothiazines and tricyclic anti-depressants. It may also be found in association with electrolyte disturbances such as hypokalaemia and hypomagnesaemia.

In this rhythm the beats originate in an unstable part of the ventricular myocardium. The onset may be sudden with rapid deterioration in tissue perfusion. This rhythm will degenerate into ventricular fibrillation.

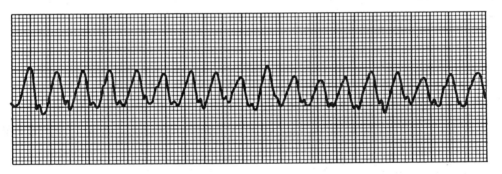

Figure 10.3. Ventricular tachycardia

Is the rate too slow?

Bradycardia is most usually a pre-terminal rhythm. It is often irregular in rhythm. Bradycardia is the final response to profound hypoxia and acidosis and its presence is ominous.

Sinus bradycardia (Figure 10.4) is an abnormally slow heart rate with a P wave of normal axis before every QRS complex. Rates below 100/min in newborns, 80/min in infants, or 60/min in older children are abnormally slow. Sinus bradycardia may occur secondary to congenital anomalies, systemic illness, or following cardiac surgery involving the atria. Acute causes include abdominal distension, increased intracranial pressure, endotracheal intubation, suctioning, and drug therapy with digoxin, β-blockers, and verapamil. In some fit adolescents sinus bradycardia may be normal.

Idioventricular rhythm occurs when the ventricle takes over the pacemaker. As the intrinsic depolarisation of the ventricles is slow the rate is usually less than 40/min.

Heart block will give rise to a regular bradycardia. Heart block may be a congenital disease or acquired following cardiac surgery.

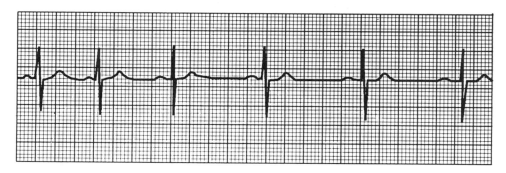

Figure 10.4. Sinus bradycardia during suctioning

In *bradycardia* it is important to note the relationship of the P and QRS complexes and the P–R interval. The QRS will be narrow or wide depending on where the pacemaker is located.

Are the complexes narrow or wide?

Narrow complexes arise when the pacemaker lies in the atria, so a supraventricular tachycardia usually shows regular narrow complexes. A regular broad QRS complex can develop due to some forms of aberrant conduction, but this is rare.

Wide complexes arise when the pacemaker lies in the ventricles. This is because conduction occurs directly through the myocardium, rather than through the fast conducting system.

Arrhythmia management

Treatment will depend on the rate, rhythm, and complex type. *Most importantly, it will depend on whether the child is stable or in cardiogenic shock.*

The pulse rate, BP, Sao_2 (percentage oxygen saturation of arterial blood), and cardiac rhythm should be monitored continuously.

An intravenous or intraosseous line should be established, although direct current (DC) shock should not be delayed for this in the pulseless or shocked patient.

Sinus tachycardia

This requires no specific treatment. The heart rate will fall with appropriate treatment of the underlying illness.

Stable supraventricular tachycardia

If the child is not in shock try vagal stimulation while continuing ECG monitoring. The following techniques can be used:

1. Elicit the "diving reflex" which produces an increase in vagal tone, slows atrioventricular conduction and interrupts the tachycardia. In the case of a baby, the infant should be wrapped in a towel and his whole face immersed in iced water for about 5 seconds. There is no need to obstruct the mouth or nostrils as the baby will be temporarily apnoeic. For an older child an ice-water soaked cloth is placed on the nose and mouth.
2. One-sided carotid body massage.
3. Older children can try a Valsalva manoeuvre. Some children know that a certain position or action will usually effect a return to sinus rhythm.

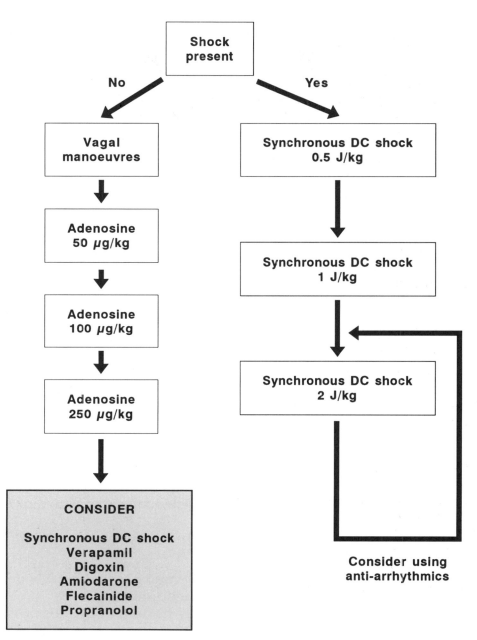

Figure 10.5. Algorithm for the management of supraventricular tachycardia

If these manoeuvres are unsuccessful consider using one of the following:

- Intravenous adenosine: start with a bolus dose of 50 µg/kg intravenously and increase the dose by 50 µg/kg after 2 minutes if success is not achieved. The next dose should be 250 µg/kg. The maximum total dose that should be given is 500 µg/kg. Adenosine is a very rapidly acting drug with a half-life of less than 10 seconds. This means that side effects (flushing, nausea, dyspnoea, chest tightness) are short-lived. It also means, however, that the effect may be shortlasting and the supraventricular tachycardia may be re-established. For the same reason if the drug is given through a small peripheral vein, an insufficiently high concentration may reach the heart and therefore a larger dose may need to be given. Adenosine is the drug of choice for supraventricular tachycardia because of its efficacy and safety record.

If a child with stable supraventricular tachycardia has not been converted to a normal rhythm with intravenous adenosine it is essential to seek the advice of a paediatric cardiologist.

- Verapamil: this drug has been associated with irreversible hypotension and asystole when given to infants. It therefore should *not be used in children under 1 year of age.* The dose for 1–5 years is 15 μg/kg intravenously slowly, from 5 to 10 years 50 μg/kg, from 10 to 15 years 100 μg/kg. The drug should be terminated when sinus rhythm is seen even though the calculated dose has not been given. *Do not use if a patient has received β-blockers.*
- Digoxin 30 μg/kg intramuscularly in three divided doses over the first 24 hours and then 4 μg/kg every 12 hours, maximum 250 μg/dose.
- Amiodarone: this drug can be used in refractory atrial tachycardia. The dose is 5 mg/kg over 20–120 min diluted in approximately 4 ml/kg of 5% dextrose.
- Flecainide 2 mg/kg over 20 minutes: this drug is particularly useful in refractory Wolff–Parkinson–White-type tachycardia. It is a membrane stabiliser but can be pro-arrhythmic and has a negative inotropic effect.
- Propranolol 100 μg/kg *slowly* intravenously: only if pacing is available as asystole may occur. *Do not give propranolol if the patient has been given verapamil.*

Unstable supraventricular tachycardia

If the child is in shock use synchronised direct current (DC) shock, 0·5–1·0 J/kg body weight/shock. If this is ineffective, increase the shock to 2 J/kg. However, recurrence of the arrhythmia should be treated with the initial dose following the administration of a pharmacological agent as discussed above.

Intravenous adenosine is rather like giving a "medical shock" and is used in preference to electrical shock in some centres. However, there should be no delay while attempting to establish an intravenous line to give this treatment in preference to DC shock. The management of supraventricular tachycardia is shown in Figure 10.5.

Ventricular tachycardia

If shock is not present, give lignocaine 0·5–1 mg/kg as an intravenous bolus dose followed by an infusion at 10–50 μg/kg body weight/minute.

If this drug is ineffectual then amiodarone may be used in the dose given above. An alternative (which is especially effective in the resistant ventricular tachycardia of tricyclic antidepressant toxicity) is phenytoin. Phenytoin should be used in a dose of 18 mg/kg over 30 minutes.

Unstable ventricular tachycardia

First ensure patent, protected airway and effective ventilation with oxygen. Give a non-synchronised DC shock of 0·5–1·0 J/kg followed by a bolus and subsequent infusion of intravenous lignocaine. If lignocaine is ineffectual then amiodarone or phenytoin may be used as above. The management of ventricular tachycardia is shown in Figure 10.6.

Wide complex tachycardia

Although 95% of narrow complex tachycardias are supraventricular in children, occasionally a wide complex tachycardia may be supraventricular in origin. Adenosine can be used to distinguish the origin of a tachycardia in a stable patient. Unstable patients should be treated as if they had ventricular tachycardia. The management of wide complex tachycardia is shown in Figure 10.7.

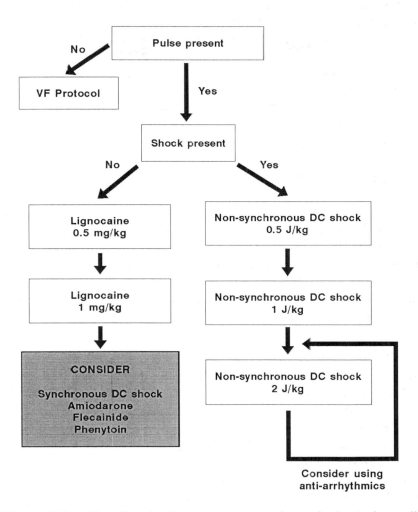

Figure 10.6. Algorithm for the management of ventricular tachycardia

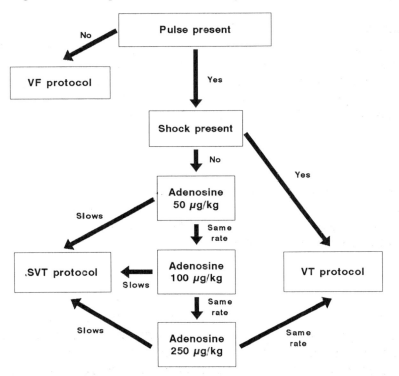

Figure 10.7. Algorithm for the management of wide complex tachycardia

Bradycardia

In paediatric practice bradycardia is almost always a pre-terminal finding in patients with respiratory or circulatory insufficiency. Airway, breathing, and circulation should always be assessed and treated if necessary before pharmacological management of bradycardia.

Bradycardia in an unstable newborn

Treat initially by supporting ventilation with oxygen and chest compressions. If these measures are not effective adrenaline 10 μg/kg intravenously is given (see Chapter 8). Atropine is ineffective in this age group.

Bradycardia in an unstable child

Treat hypoxia and shock with intubation, ventilation, and volume expansion. If these measures do not lead to rapid improvement, consider a bolus of adrenaline 10 μg/kg intravenously followed by an adrenaline or isoprenaline infusion. The dose of adrenaline for infusion is 1–2 μg/kg/min. The dose for isoprenaline is 0·02–0·2 μg/kg/min. Atropine 0·02 mg/kg intravenously (minimum dose 0·1 mg, maximum 2·0 mg/dose) may be of benefit. If there is still no improvement consider cardiac pacing.

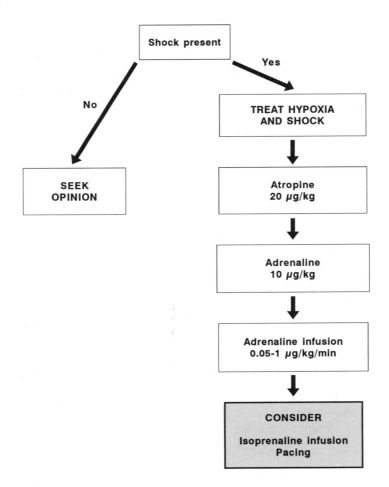

Figure 10.8. Algorithm for the management of bradycardia

CARDIOGENIC SHOCK

Cardiogenic shock may occur because of mechanical or physiological problems within the heart itself. Examples include myocarditis, cardiomyopathies, congenital malformations, and arrhythmias. Alternatively, the function of the myocardium may be impaired as a result of systemic disturbances such as hypoxia, acidosis, and toxins (endogenous as in septicaemia and exogenous as in poisonings).

Cardiogenic shock may be suspected:

1. Following cardiopulmonary resuscitation with adequate fluid replacement. The cause of cardiogenic shock is then hypoxia/ischaemia.
2. In patients with septic shock who have failed to improve despite adequate fluid replacement. Bacterial toxins are the suggested cause of cardiogenic shock in this instance.
3. In patients with a known history of heart disease who present in shock.
4. In patients who have been previously well, present in shock, and have a large heart on chest radiograph. The diagnosis of myocarditis or cardiomyopathy is likely here.
5. In patients who present in shock with a history of ingesting a poison known to damage the myocardium, e.g. tricyclic antidepressant.

The physiological responses to decreased cardiac output which are beneficial in hypovolaemic shock may be damaging in cardiogenic shock. Retention of water and sodium by the kidneys leads to an increase in extracellular fluid, circulatory congestion, and oedema. An increase in systemic vascular resistance due to the release of vasoactive substances can worsen cardiogenic shock by increasing the afterload on a poorly contractile myocardium. Furthermore, hypoxia and acidosis lead to capillary stasis, decreased venous return, and a reduction in the effective circulating blood volume.

Clinically, patients in cardiogenic shock may have, in addition to the usual features of shock (as described in Chapter 9), evidence of circulatory overload with jugular venous distension, hepatomegaly, pulmonary oedema, and gallop rhythm.

Therapeutic measures

Treatment is directed as follows.

Treatment to increase oxygen supply and delivery
- Give high-flow oxygen by bag and mask.
- Consider mechanical ventilation with positive end-expiratory pressure (PEEP), especially if pulmonary oedema is present.
- Correct anaemia with slow infusion of packed cells if haemoglobin is below 10 g.
- If haemoglobin is very low (<5 g) an exchange transfusion should be performed.

Treatment to decrease oxygen requirements
- Treat hypothermia with external heat and insulation: treat hyperthermia by cooling and antipyretics.
- Relieve pain.
- Mechanical ventilation may be required if the work of breathing is excessive.

Optimise preload
- Insert a central venous pressure line to assess fluid requirements.
- Carefully infuse colloid in aliquots of 10 ml/kg. If central venous pressure exceeds

10 mmHg and there is no improvement in cardiac output then further increase in preload would be harmful.

- If there is vascular congestion (shown clinically by peripheral oedema and crepitations, radiologically, or a sustained rise of central venous pressure), then intravenous diuretics will be needed, e.g. frusemide 1 mg/kg.

Reduce afterload

- Relieve pain.
- Sedate if ventilation is supported.
- Give vasodilators (see below).

Improve myocardial contractility

- Improvement in oxygenation will help myocardial contractility.
- Correct metabolic abnormalities, such as acidosis, hypoglycaemia, and electrolyte disturbances.
- Give inotropic drug support (see below).

Inotropic drugs

Catecholamines are the most potent inotropes, but have complex chronotropic effects and alter the vascular bed. The choice of drug depends on the state of the circulation as much as on the state of the myocardium. Catecholamines commonly used are dopamine, dobutamine, adrenaline, isoprenaline, and noradrenaline.

Although they are used extensively, the dose response of catecholamines is not fully documented and therefore they must be monitored very carefully in use.

Dopamine Dopamine acts both directly on cardiac β-adrenergic receptors, and indirectly through the release of noradrenaline. As it is dependent on the patient's noradrenaline stores for part of its action, it may be ineffective in children with chronic cardiac conditions and the very young. In low doses (5–10 µg/kg/min), dopamine produces vasodilatation and increased blood flow in the kidneys. Dopamine is often used in this way together with dobutamine. The two drugs will augment myocardial contractility and maintain renal blood flow. In higher doses (10–20 µg/kg/min), the main action of dopamine is to increase heart rate and blood pressure from peripheral vasoconstriction.

Dobutamine Dobutamine is a direct-acting catecholamine which does not depend on endogenous noradrenaline. It can therefore be more effective in patients in cardiogenic shock. Dobutamine increases cardiac output by increasing cardiac contractility and heart rate, but has little effect on peripheral vascular tone. It is less effective in infants.

Isoprenaline Isoprenaline is a β-adrenergic agonist. It increases heart rate and myocardial contractility. It also produces peripheral and skeletal muscle vasodilatation. Attention must therefore be given to ensuring that circulating volume is adequate. Isoprenaline is a useful inotrope in children under the age of 1 year with cardiogenic shock. It may also be useful in patients with unstable bradycardia due to heart block where atropine has been ineffective.

Adrenaline Adrenaline is a very potent adrenergic inotrope. It will increase heart rate, myocardial contractility, and increase peripheral vascular resistance. The indication for adrenaline infusion is failure of other inotropes, most particularly in the young infant or child with chronic heart disease. It may cause severe peripheral vasoconstriction and arrhythmias.

96

Precautions All inotropes can cause a marked increase in heart rate and cause tachyarrhythmias. They should preferably be given through a central venous line as peripheral infusion, and particularly extravasation of the infusion, can result in severe local tissue damage. The drugs may be diluted in saline or dextrose solutions. They are inactivated by sodium bicarbonate.

> **Never flush through an intravenous catheter with inotropic drugs in it; rapid administration could be fatal**
> **Never interrupt the infusion of inotropic drugs as the half-life is very short**
> **All drug infusions must be labelled accurately with the name, concentration, diluent, and rate**

Vasodilators

These drugs are most effective where there is raised peripheral resistance. They increase the vascular bed. Caution must be observed when using these drugs and a central venous pressure monitor is mandatory. Hypotension and poor myocardial perfusion can result from too rapid vasodilatation.

Arteriolar dilatation results in an increased ejection fraction, increased stroke volume, and decreased end-systolic left ventricular volume. Venous dilatation leads to a shift of blood into the peripheral circulation, and reduced right and left ventricular diastolic volume. This benefits both the pulmonary and the systemic capillary pressures leading to a reduction in oedema by decreased myocardial wall stress and improved diastolic perfusion of the myocardium.

Sodium nitroprusside This is a balanced arterial and venous dilator. It may result in cyanide toxicity after a few days' use. Doses of more than $5 \mu g/kg/min$ may result in decreased urine output because of change in renal blood flow.

Nitroglycerin This is a venous dilator but the dose is not well established in young children and infants.

> **Important considerations when using drugs in the treatment of shock**
>
> - Initial management is with fluids
> - The main aim of therapy is to restore tissue perfusion
> - Both inotropes and vasodilators are very powerful groups of drugs with quantitatively unpredictable effects. They should be used ideally only in patients who have full circulatory monitoring in a paediatric intensive care unit. In a seriously ill, non-invasively monitored child, however, inotropes may be needed urgently. Dopamine and/or dobutamine are suitable for use in this situation. In a desperate case an adrenaline infusion may be used but transfer for monitoring should be arranged as soon as possible

Enoximone This is an inhibitor of intravenous phosphodiesterase. It prevents the inactivation of cyclic AMP. It increases cardiac output without chronotropic effects and reduces preload and afterload of the heart. Enoximone has some inotropic effect.

These tests are required to assess the patient's needs and monitor treatment:

- ECG monitor.
- Blood pressure:
    initially by non-invasive method;
    as soon as possible establish an arterial line for continuous pressure monitoring and arterial blood gas sampling.

97

- Pulse oximetry.
- Peripheral intravenous infusion in situ.
- Core/skin temperature differential.
- As soon as possible establish a central venous line to monitor central venous pressure and give inotropic drugs, sodium bicarbonate, etc.

Table 10.1. Commonly used cardiovascular drugs in shock

Drug	Dose (μg/kg/min)	Notes
Dopamine	1–20	α-, β-Adrenergic and dopaminergic effects Cardiovascular effects are dose dependent When used in low dose ($< 10 \mu$g/kg/min) can restore contractility and improve renal function
Dobutamine	1–20	α-, β-Adrenergic effects Inotropic effect with minimal increased heart rate or increased systemic vascular resistance
Adrenaline	0·05–1·0	α-, β-Adrenergic effects Dose-related response High dose leads to marked vasoconstriction Useful to help maintain cardiac output and BP in children in whom dopamine+dobutamine is unsuccessful
Isoprenaline	0·05–0·5	Marked chronotropic effect Useful in bradycardia not responsive to atropine Causes vasodilatation
Noradrenaline	0·05–1·0	α-Adrenergic effect Very powerful vasoconstrictor, used when other inotropes and fluid therapy are unsuccessful Very similar to adrenaline
Vasodilators Nitroglycerin	0·5–20	Venous dilator
Nitroprusside	0·05–6	Arterial and venous dilator Can cause cyanide poisoning
Enoximone	5–20	Arterial vasodilator

Summary of treatment of cardiogenic shock

1. Give 100% oxygen via a face-mask. In a critically ill patient, or if there is pulmonary oedema, intubate immediately and start intermittent positive pressure ventilation (IPPV).
2. Treat hypotension with plasma 10 ml/kg stat. Repeat if required. Monitoring of central venous pressure is necessary to assess volume requirements.
3. Correct acid/base status with sodium bicarbonate based on arterial blood gas results if the pH is below 7·15. These patients should be ventilated.
4. Correct any electrolyte imbalance and hypoglycaemia.
5. Support failing myocardium with inotropes:
   - dopamine (5–10 μg/kg/min)
   - ±dobutamine (5–10 μg/kg/min)
   - or adrenaline (0·5–1 μg/kg/min)
   - or isoprenaline (0·05–0·5 μg/kg/min)
6. Reduce afterload:
   - nitroprusside (0·05–8 μg/kg/min)
   - or enoximone (5–20 μg/kg/min)
7. Maintain urine output to at least 1 ml/kg/h, with:
   - volume expansion
   - diuretics
   - dopamine infusion

MANAGEMENT OF THE INFANT WITH A DUCT-DEPENDENT CONGENITAL HEART DISEASE

There are several complex congenital heart defects in which the presence of a patent ductus arteriosus is essential to maintain pulmonary or systemic flow. The normal patent ductus arteriosus closes functionally in the first 24 hours of life. This may be delayed in the presence of congenital cardiac abnormalities. With modern obstetric management many babies are now discharged from the maternity unit only hours after birth. Therefore babies with serious congenital neonatal heart disease may present to paediatric or accident and emergency departments.

The pulmonary obstructive lesions include pulmonary atresia, critical pulmonary valve stenosis, tricuspid atresia, severe Fallot's tetralogy, and some cases of transposition of the great vessels. In all of these lesions there is no effective exit for blood from the right ventricle into the pulmonary circulation, and therefore pulmonary blood flow and oxygenation of blood are dependent on flow from the aorta via a patent ductus.

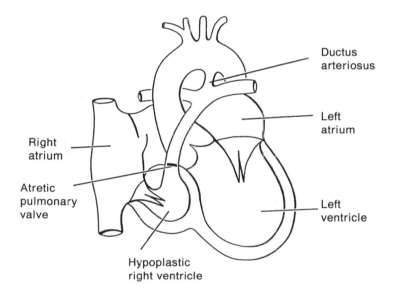

Figure 10.9. Pulmonary outflow obstruction

Babies with critical pulmonary obstructive lesions present in the first few days of life with increasing cyanosis, breathlessness, or cardiogenic shock. On examination there may be a characteristic murmur but in fact more frequently there is no murmur audible. An enlarged liver is a common finding. The clinical situation has arisen from the gradual closure of the ductus arteriosus. Complete closure will result in the death of the infant from hypoxia.

Additionally, there are some congenital heart malformations where systemic blood flow is dependent on the ductus arteriosus delivering blood to the aorta and the pulmonary circulation. This is characteristic of severe coarctation, critical aortic stenosis, and hypoplastic left heart syndrome.

In these congenital heart lesions the baby ceases to be able to feed and becomes breathless, grey, and collapsed with a poor peripheral circulation. On examination the babies are in heart failure and in more severe cases in cardiogenic shock. In this situation, even in coarctation of the aorta, all pulses are difficult to feel.

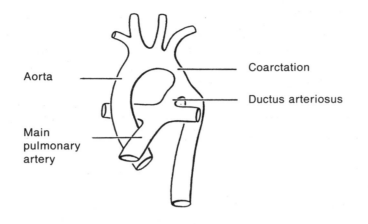

Figure 10.10. Aortic coarctation

The treatment of both of these groups of duct-dependent congenital heart disease is the same. An infusion of prostaglandin E_2 at a dose of $0.05\ \mu g/kg/min$ will maintain or increase the patent ductus arteriosus size temporarily until the patient can be transferred to a neonatal cardiology unit. Patients should be intubated and ventilated for transfer both because of the seriousness of their condition and also because the prostaglandin may cause apnoea.

It is also important to avoid hypothermia, correct hypoglycaemia, hypocalcaemia, or hypovolaemia and correct acid–base disturbances based on arterial blood gas indications. A high concentration of oxygen is clearly not helpful. Oxygen concentration for ventilation should be individually adjusted using pulse oximetry to monitor the most effective concentration for each infant.

ACUTE PULMONARY OUTFLOW TRACT OBSTRUCTION (CYANOTIC ATTACKS)

Patients with Fallot's tetralogy can sometimes develop a sudden increase in the right ventricular outflow tract obstruction caused by spasm of the infundibulum. This prevents right ventricular blood from reaching the lungs and therefore it flows into the aorta causing severe systemic hypoxia. The child looks more blue or may become very pale. He will usually lose consciousness and may have convulsions. Attacks are often self-limiting but some children may die during an attack or suffer the effects of cerebral anoxia.

Treatment is to provide high concentration face-mask oxygen and to give morphine $25\ \mu g/kg$ intramuscularly. If this is ineffective intravenous propranolol $100\ \mu g/kg$ will usually result in improvement.

SYSTEMIC HYPERTENSIVE CRISIS

Hypertension is uncommon in children. Blood pressure is rarely measured routinely in otherwise healthy children and therefore hypertension usually presents with symptoms. Neurological symptoms are more common in children than in adults. Children may present with hypertensive encephalopathy. Symptoms will include severe headaches and vomiting which are indicative of raised intracranial pressure or with coma or convulsions. Some children will present with facial palsy or a hemiplegia.

Accelerated hypertension is defined as a blood pressure greater than the 95th percentile for age and sex in which there is evidence of end-organ dysfunction such as hypertensive retinopathy. The blood pressure measurement should be repeated several times and the correct cuff size must be used.

Most children with raised blood pressure have secondary hypertension. The most common causes are renal followed by vascular abnormalities such as coarctation of the aorta or abnormalities of the renal artery. Endocrine causes of such a phaeochromocytoma are rare.

In the treatment of a hypertensive emergency the aim must be for slow reduction of blood pressure. There is ample evidence that rapid reduction of blood pressure in a hypertensive child causes a high incidence of permanent neurological sequelae. The aim should be to bring the blood pressure down to the 95th percentile for age (120 systolic at age 5 years, 130 systolic at age 12 years) over 3–4 days. In the first 24 hours the aim should be to reduce the blood pressure by only a third of the desired reduction. Some children may be anuric; urea, electrolytes, and creatinine should be analysed promptly.

The currently recommended drugs to achieve blood pressure reduction in children include the following alternatives:

- Labetolol 1–3 mg/kg/h.
- Sodium nitroprusside 0·5–6 µg/kg/min.

The dose should be titrated in increments according to the child's blood pressure. If there is a fall greater than the lower limit that has been set for that child then normal or physiological saline should be administered in boluses of 50 ml to keep the blood pressure at the desired level. Blood pressure should be measured at 5-minute intervals while the infusion is running, and at 15-minute intervals when it is temporarily discontinued.

These children require intensive monitoring and nursing. Therefore, if a child presents with severe hypertension, treatment should be delayed until after discussion with a paediatric nephrologist or cardiologist. Some may recommend the use of sublingual nifedipine as a temporary measure before transfer; if any drug is used the child should have the blood pressure monitored as above and an intravenous infusion in place.

In a child presenting with a life-threatening complication such as raised intracranial pressure, supportive ventilation and diuretic therapy should be started as usual, while seeking urgent expert advice. Such children may have had a cerebral haemorrhage.

HEART FAILURE

Aetiology

In infancy heart failure is usually secondary to structural heart disease and medical treatment is directed to improving the clinical condition prior to definitive surgery. In the older child myocarditis and cardiomyopathy are the most common underlying disorders (see box).

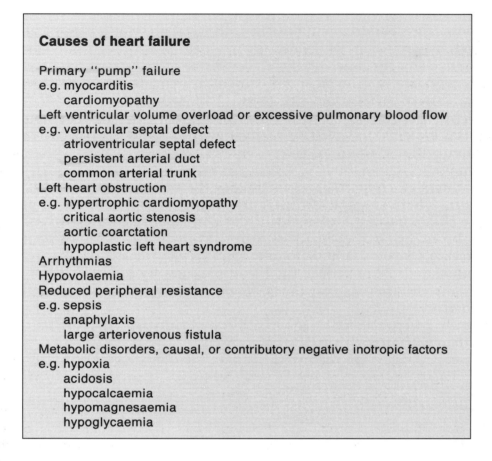

Causes of heart failure

Primary "pump" failure
e.g. myocarditis
    cardiomyopathy
Left ventricular volume overload or excessive pulmonary blood flow
e.g. ventricular septal defect
    atrioventricular septal defect
    persistent arterial duct
    common arterial trunk
Left heart obstruction
e.g. hypertrophic cardiomyopathy
    critical aortic stenosis
    aortic coarctation
    hypoplastic left heart syndrome
Arrhythmias
Hypovolaemia
Reduced peripheral resistance
e.g. sepsis
    anaphylaxis
    large arteriovenous fistula
Metabolic disorders, causal, or contributory negative inotropic factors
e.g. hypoxia
    acidosis
    hypocalcaemia
    hypomagnesaemia
    hypoglycaemia

Clinical features of heart failure

The common features in infancy are breathlessness, feeding difficulty with growth failure, restlessness, and sweating. Older children may present with fatigue, effort intolerance, anorexia, abdominal pain, and cough. There is tachycardia, tachypnoea, sternal, and subcostal recession. The extremities are cool and pale with cardiomegaly and hepatomegaly. Auscultation reveals a gallop rhythm and occasionally basal crackles. In babies and children peripheral oedema is less commonly seen than in adults.

Investigations

These include full blood count, serum urea and electrolytes, calcium, glucose, and arterial blood gases. Perform a routine infection screen including blood cultures especially in infants. A full 12-lead ECG and chest radiograph are essential. All patients suspected of having structural heart disease should be discussed with a paediatric cardiologist; echocardiography will establish the diagnosis in almost all cases.

Treatment

General measures should include oxygen administration, correction of anaemia, acidosis, and metabolic abnormalities. Hypovolaemia should be corrected by appropriate volume infusion. If infection is likely broad-spectrum antibiotics should be given. Cardiac arrhythmia requires prompt correct diagnosis and control. If duct-dependent systemic circulation is likely, emergency intravenous administration of prostaglandin E_2 should be commenced.

Drug treatment

Diuretics These drugs remain the mainstay of treatment for heart failure. They increase urinary sodium and water excretion, and reduce systemic and pulmonary venous congestion. They improve cardiac output by this preload reduction. Important adverse effects are hypokalaemia and hypovolaemia from excessive diuresis.

Frusemide is the most commonly used diuretic. It acts on the loop of Henle primarily inhibiting active chloride resorption. Give 1 mg/kg intravenously followed by initial maintenance dose of 1–2 mg/kg/day in one to three divided doses. If there is no diuresis within 2 hours, the intravenous bolus can be repeated (maximum 4 mg/kg/dose). Potassium supplementation or concurrent administration of a potassium-sparing agent will be required. Bumetanide (1 mg dose equivalent to 40 mg frusemide) and ethacrynic acid offer no clear advantages over frusemide.

Aldosterone antagonists act indirectly on the distal tubule sodium–potassium exchange. They increase sodium loss and correct the potassium loss produced by loop diuretics. Spironolactone is given in a dose of 1–3 mg/kg/day; alternatively amiloride (which acts directly on the distal tubule) 0·2 mg/kg/dose twice daily is effective. These drugs can result in hyperkalaemia particularly if there is impaired renal function. They should not be given in conjunction with angiotensin-converting enzyme (ACE) inhibitors.

Digoxin There has been some controversy as to the role of digoxin in the treatment of heart failure. Digitalis glycosides act via calcium-dependent sodium–potassium ATPase and increase systolic contractility. They increase cardiac output, particularly where there is impaired left ventricular function. Patients with large left-to-right shunts and high pulmonary blood flow have normal or supranormal left ventricular contractility. The use of digoxin in this group is therefore theoretically open to question, though in practice digoxin is beneficial in infants with left-to-right shunts and still widely used.

Digitalis glycosides slow atrioventricular conduction and unequivocally are effective when heart failure is associated with atrial arrhythmias and rapid ventricular rates. They reduce ventricular rate, and consequently increase ventricular filling and cardiac output.

Digoxin has a narrow therapeutic range. Toxicity is exacerbated by hypokalaemia, hypercalcaemia, and impaired renal function. Pre-term infants require lower maintenance doses than was thought necessary in the past. Intoxication results in new arrhythmias, particularly atrial tachycardias with atrioventricular block. Digoxin can be given intravenously though this should only be necessary in emergency situations where oral medication is not possible (see Table 10.2 for digitalising and maintenance doses).

The following drugs require careful haemodynamic assessment and monitoring, and should only be used after discussion with a paediatric cardiologist

Table 10.2. Digoxin dosage

Digitalising dose (µg/kg total dose over 24 hours, given in three divided doses)		Maintenance dose (µg/kg total daily dose, given in two divided doses)	
30 IV	40 oral	8 IV	8 oral

Adjust dose to maintain blood levels 1–2 µg/l (peak levels 6 hours after oral dose).

Vasodilators In cardiac failure, compensatory mechanisms that are initially beneficial can become disadvantageous. Thus increased preload, which initially augments cardiac output via the Frank–Starling mechanism, can result in symptomatic pulmonary and systemic venous congestion. As ventricular wall stress increases, myocardial oxygen requirements rise. Increased peripheral resistance may maintain systemic blood pressure, though by increasing afterload this may reduce stroke volume and cardiac output further.

Vasodilators can improve cardiac output by reducing afterload and improve symptomatic venous congestion by preload reduction. These drugs are particularly effective in heart failure secondary to cardiomyopathy, severe mitral or aortic regurgitation, myocardial ischaemia, and post-cardiac surgery. *They should not be used where preload is low as they may further reduce cardiac output. They are contraindicated where heart failure due to a fixed obstructive lesion.*

Captopril This is now the most commonly used vasodilator in children with heart failure. It is an orally active competitive inhibitor of angiotensin-converting enzyme (ACE), thereby reducing production of angiotensin II and increasing production of vasodilator bradykinin. It is a balanced arterial and venous dilator. The major adverse effect is hypotension which is exacerbated by hyponatraemia. In infants a test dose of 0·1 mg/kg is given followed by 0·1 mg/kg three times daily increasing to 0·5 mg/kg three times daily. If required this can be increased to a maximum of 2 mg/kg per dose. Rare adverse reactions are proteinuria and neutropenia. Hyperkalaemia may occur because of aldosterone antagonism and potassium-sparing diuretics should not be given in conjunction with ACE inhibitors.

Enalapril Enalapril is also an ACE inhibitor which has been used in children as an alternative to captopril. It is given in an initial dose of 0·2 mg/kg/day in two divided doses increasing, if necessary, to a maximum of 0·5 mg/kg/day. Side effects and cautions are as for captopril.

Nitrates These act predominantly to reduce preload via venous dilatation. They are not commonly used in children but can be very effective where high filling pressures accompany low cardiac output after cardiac surgery, and for the emergency treatment of pulmonary oedema secondary to severe mitral or aortic regurgitation.

Inotropic agents These agents are used in severe heart failure and cardiogenic shock. The most commonly used agents are dopamine, dobutamine, and isoprenaline. They all require intensive haemodynamic monitoring and intravenous administration.

CHAPTER
11

Convulsions (status epilepticus)

Definitions

Convulsion or seizure
This is an abnormal paroxysmal discharge of cerebral neurones.

Status epilepticus
This occurs either when a convulsion lasts for longer than 30 minutes or when successive convulsions occur so frequently that the patient does not recover fully between them.

Tonic–clonic status is the most common form of status epilepticus. It occurs in approximately 1–5% of patients with epilepsy. Five to ten per cent of children with febrile seizures will present in status epilepticus.

The mortality associated with status epilepticus is 3–20%. Mortality is higher in adults. Death may be due to complications of the convulsion, such as obstruction of the airway or aspiration of vomit, to over-medication, or to the underlying disease process.

PATHOPHYSIOLOGY

Injury to the brain during status epilepticus occurs as a result of one of the following:

- The underlying disease, e.g. meningitis.
- Systemic complications of the convulsions, especially hypoxia from airway obstruction, and later acidosis when systemic hypotension occurs.
- Direct injury from repetitive neuronal discharge.

A generalised convulsion increases the cerebral metabolic rate at least threefold. Initially, there is an increased sympathetic activity with release of catecholamines which lead to peripheral vasoconstriction and increased systemic blood pressure. There is also loss of cerebral arterial regulation and, following the increase in systemic blood pressure, there is a resulting increase in cerebral blood flow to provide the necessary oxygen and energy. If convulsions continue, the systemic blood pressure falls and this is followed by a fall in cerebral blood flow. The energy requirements of the brain fall, lactic acid accumulates and there is subsequently cell death, oedema, and raised intracerebral pressure resulting in further worsening of cerebral perfusion. Cellular metabolism of calcium and sodium is also impaired with further cell death.

Approximately two-thirds of children with status epilepticus that lasts longer than 60 minutes will have irreversible neurological handicaps. The incidence of neurological complications is higher in young infants – and status is far more common in this age group.

Most common causes of status epilepticus in children

"Febrile" status epilepticus
Sudden reduction in anti-epileptic medication
Acute cerebral trauma
Idiopathic epilepsy
Bacterial meningitis
Encephalopathy (including Reye's syndrome)
Poisoning

MANAGEMENT

Airway and breathing

- Establish airway and ensure adequate oxygenation and ventilation. Give 100% oxygen; suck out the oropharynx as necessary.
- Use bag-and-mask ventilation if the patient is hypoxic or not ventilating adequately. Rarely, it is necessary to proceed to intubation at this stage. An anaesthetist should perform this because rapid sequence induction will be necessary.

Circulation

Check the blood glucose and establish intravenous access. Give intravenous glucose (0·5 g/kg as 25% solution) if the blood glucose is below 3 mmol/l. If there is no evidence of shock give minimal (2–3 ml/kg/h) isotonic fluid to minimise the risk of cerebral oedema.

Anticonvulsant drug therapy

Follow the protocol in Figure 11.1.

Diazepam
Dose: 0·25–0·4 mg/kg intravenous bolus given over 30–40 seconds; 0·5 mg/kg per rectum; 100–400 µg/kg/h by infusion.
This is an effective, quick-acting anticonvulsant, which works within 5–10 minutes but whose action is short lasting (about 40 minutes to 1 hour). It has a depressant effect on respiration and this is enhanced by the addition of other anticonvulsants such as phenobarbitone. Also, repeated doses make side effects more marked. The rectal dose is well absorbed and acts almost as quickly as the intravenous dose.

Paraldehyde
Dose: 0·4 ml/kg per rectum, made up as a 50:50 solution in arachis oil. This can cause rectal irritation, but intramuscular paraldehyde causes severe pain and may lead to sterile abscess formation.

106

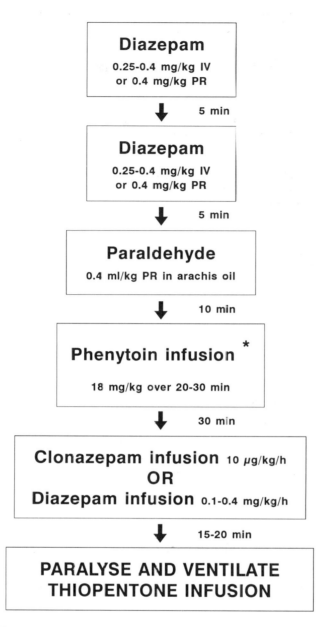

Figure 11.1. Treatment protocol for status epilepticus.
* Unless already on phenytoin regularly – use paraldehyde.

Paraldehyde causes little respiratory depression. It should not be used in liver disease. Paraldehyde takes 10–15 minutes to act and its action is sustained for 2–4 hours.

Do not leave paraldehyde standing in a plastic syringe for longer than a few minutes.

Phenytoin

Dose: 18 mg/kg intravenously over 20–30 minutes. Rate of infusion no greater than 1 mg/kg/min. Infusion to be made up in 0·9% sodium chloride solution to a maximum concentration of 1 mg in 1 ml.

Measure plasma phenytoin levels 90–120 minutes after the completion of the infusion.

Phenytoin can cause dysrhythmias and hypotension, and therefore an ECG monitor should be used and the BP monitored. It has little depressant effect on respiration.

Do not use this if the child is known to be on oral phenytoin until the blood level of phenytoin is known. Then only give it if the phenytoin level is less than 2·5 µg/ml. Phenytoin has a peak action within 1 hour but a long half-life that is dose dependent. Its action therefore is more sustained than diazepam and it is useful in status epilepticus.

Thiopentone sodium

Induction dose 4–8 mg/kg intravenously.

This is an alkaline solution which will cause irritation if the solution leaks into subcutaneous tissues.

It has no analgesic effect and is a general anaesthetic agent. Repeated doses have a cumulative effect. It is a potent drug with marked cardiorespiratory effects and should be used only by experienced staff who can intubate a child.

It is not an effective long-term anticonvulsant and its principal use in status epilepticus is to facilitate ventilation and the subsequent management of cerebral oedema due to the prolonged seizure activity. Other anti-epileptic medication must be continued. A baseline EEG should be obtained as soon as possible after the child has been paralysed and ventilated.

Clonazepam

Dose: infusion of 10 µg/kg/h.

This anticonvulsant can cause hypersalivation and hypotonia. It has a marked respiratory depressant effect and should be used under specialist supervision, preferably in intensive care.

Alternative regimens

Alternative anticonvulsant infusion regimens are available, but should only be tried if there is a recurrence of seizures after initial control of status, and despite maximum rates of infusion of either diazepam or clonazepam.

In decreasing order of preference the alternative regimens are:

- Chlormethiazole (0·8% solution containing 8 mg/ml), commencing at 8 mg/kg/h. This should be given in an A-2001 administration set which should be changed every 12 hours.
- Paraldehyde 1–4 ml/kg/h of 5% solution.
- Lignocaine: initial loading dose of 5 mg/kg intravenously; infusion rate of 3–6 mg/kg/h.

General measures

Fluid input should be kept to 50–60% normal requirements, using 0·45% saline and 5% dextrose. Monitoring includes pulse, blood pressure, respiratory rate, oxygen saturation, urine output, blood levels of glucose, urea, creatinine and electrolytes. The role of cerebral function analysis monitoring (CFAM) is still unclear. At the current time clinical features and standard EEG are the preferred method of assessing seizure activity.

Additional treatments will depend on the clinical situation.

Frequent reassessment of ABC is mandatory as therapy may cause depression of ventilation or hypotension.

In the child with a core temperature of > 39°C give rectal paracetamol.

INVESTIGATIONS

Mandatory investigations

- Glucose.
- Calcium.
- Phosphate.

- Magnesium.
- Full blood count.
- Urine and electrolytes.
- Arterial blood gas.

Optional investigations (depending on history and examination)

- Toxicology.
- Septic screen (for contraindications to lumbar puncture, see Chapter 10).
- Ammonia.
- Liver function tests.
- Metabolic screening.
- Clotting screen.
- Chest radiograph.
- Computed tomography (CT) scan.

Monitor

- ECG.
- Blood pressure.
- Pulse oximetry.
- Core temperature.
- Urine output.

Other medical complications, which are infrequently associated with status epilepticus and which usually follow prolonged status, include cardiac dysrhythmias, pulmonary oedema, disseminated intravascular coagulation, myoglobinuria, and hyperthermia.

CHAPTER

12

Coma

The conscious level may be altered by disease, injury, or intoxication. The level of awareness decreases as a child passes through stages from drowsiness (mild reduction in alertness and increase in hours of sleep) to unconsciousness (unrousable unresponsiveness). Because of variability in the definition of words describing the degree of coma, the Glasgow and the Children's Coma Scales have been developed as semiquantitative measures and, more importantly, as a communication aid between carers. The Glasgow Coma Scale has been validated whereas the Children's Coma Scale has not.

Table 12.1. Glasgow Coma Scale and Children's Coma Scale

Glasgow Coma Scale (4–15 years)		Children's Coma Scale (< 4 years)		
Response	Score	Response		Score
Eyes		Eyes		
Open spontaneously	4	Open spontaneously		4
Verbal command	3	React to speech		3
Pain	2	React to pain		2
No response	1	No response		1
Best motor response		Best motor response		
Verbal command:		Spontaneous or obeys verbal		
obeys	6	command		6
Painful stimulus:		*Painful stimulus:*		
Localises pain	5	Localises pain		5
Flexion with pain	4	Withdraws in response to pain		4
		Abnormal flexion to pain		
Flexion abnormal	3	(decorticate posture)		3
		Abnormal extension to pain		
Extension	2	(decerebrate posture)		2
No response	1	No response		1
Best verbal response		Best verbal response		
Orientated and		Smiles, orientated to sounds,		
converses	5	follows objects, interacts		5
Disorientated and		*Crying*	*Interacts*	
converses	4	Consolable	Inappropriate	4
		Inconsistently		
Inappropriate words	3	consolable	Moaning	3
Incomprehensible				
sounds	2	Inconsolable	Irritable	2
No response	1	No response	No response	1

PATHOPHYSIOLOGY AND AETIOLOGY

Coma is a sign of significant "brain failure" and requires emergency treatment to prevent or minimise central nervous system damage.

In children, coma is caused by a diffuse metabolic insult (including cerebral hypoxia and ischaemia) in 95% of cases, and by structural lesions in the remaining 5%. Metabolic disturbances can produce diffuse, incomplete, and asymmetrical neurological signs. Early signs of metabolic encephalopathy may be subtle with reduced attention and blunted affect. The most common causes of coma are summarised in the box.

Disorders causing coma in children

Hypoxic – ischaemic brain injury
  Following respiratory or circulatory failure
Epileptic seizures
Trauma
  Intracranial haemorrhage, brain swelling
Infections
   Meningitis
   Encephalitis
Poisons
Metabolic
  Renal, hepatic failure, Reye's syndrome, hypoglycaemia, diabetes, hypothermia, hypercapnia
Vascular lesions
  Bleeding, arteriovenous malformations, arterial or venous thrombosis
Hypertension

Cerebral perfusion pressure

The initial priority in the management of the unconscious child is the maintenance of adequate airway breathing, circulation, and metabolic homoeostasis. Once this has been done, attention may then be given to the possibility of raised intracranial pressure and its effects.

In very young children, before the cranial sutures are closed, considerable expansion in the intracranial volume may occur if the process is slow. However, if the process is rapid and in children with a fixed-volume cranium, increase in volume due to brain swelling, haematoma, or cerebral spinal fluid (CSF) blockage will cause raised intracranial pressure (ICP). Initially cerebrospinal fluid and venous blood within the cranium decrease in volume. Soon, this compensating mechanism fails and as the intracranial pressure continues to rise the cerebral perfusion pressure (CPP) falls and arterial blood flow is reduced.

$$CPP = MAP - ICP$$

where MAP is mean arterial pressure. Reduced CPP reduces cerebral blood flow (CBF). Normal CBF is over 50 ml/100 g brain tissue/min. If the CBF falls below 20, the brain suffers ischaemia.

Increasing intracranial pressure will push brain tissue against more rigid intracranial structures. Two clinical syndromes are recognisable by the site of localised brain compression.

Central syndrome
The whole brain is pressed down towards the foramen magnum and the cerebellar tonsils herniate through it ("coning"). Neck stiffness may be noted. A slow pulse, raised blood pressure, and irregular respiration leading to apnoea are seen terminally.

112

Uncal syndrome

The intracranial volume increase is mainly in the supratentorial part of the intracranial space. The uncus, which is part of the hippocampal gyrus, is forced through the tentorial opening and compressed against the fixed free edge of the tentorium. If the pressure is unilateral (for example, from a subdural or extradural haematoma), this leads to third nerve compression and an ipsilateral dilated pupil. Next, an external oculomotor palsy appears, so the eye cannot move laterally. Hemiplegia may then develop on either or both sides of the body, depending on the progression of the herniation.

Further signs that may be indicative of raised intracranial pressure are discussed below under "Assessment and management".

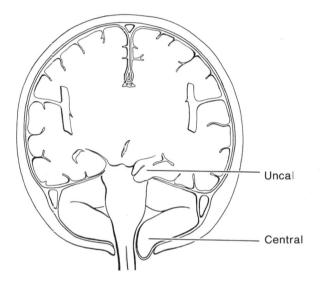

Figure 12.1. Herniations of the brain

ASSESSMENT AND MANAGEMENT

This must be sequential and methodical. Every effort should be made both to prevent secondary brain damage from hypoxia or ischaemia, from hypoglycaemia or from infection, and to minimise increased intracranial pressure.

Primary assessment and management

In the *primary* phase, airway, breathing, and circulation are assessed and stabilised. Urgent problems such as hypoglycaemia, sepsis, and raised intracranial pressure are addressed.

Airway
Establish and maintain an adequate airway.

Breathing
Give high-flow oxygen. Intubation and ventilatory support will be needed under the following conditions:

- Breathing is inadequate.
- There is no protective cough reflex or gag reflex.

113

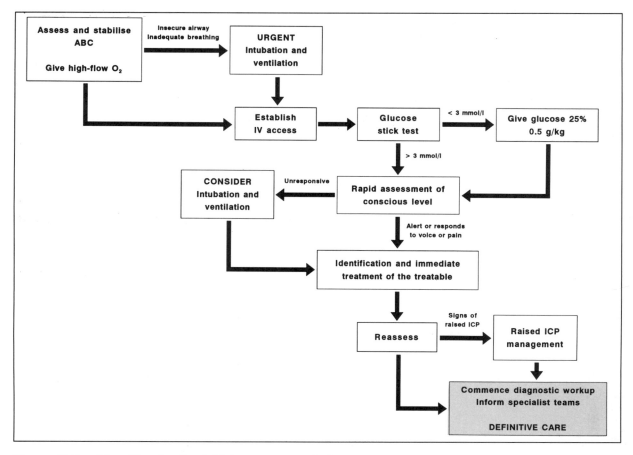

Figure 12.2. Algorithm for the initial management of coma

- The Glasgow Coma Score is less than 8.
- There are signs of impending herniation (see above).

Circulation

Establish intravenous access. If there is evidence of shock treat as in Chapter 9. In the absence of shock there should be fluid restriction (2 ml/kg/h). If significant hypertension is present this should be treated (see Chapter 10).

Hypoglycaemia

Check blood sugar with a rapid bedside stick test. Treat hypoglycaemia (<3 mmol/l) with 10% glucose 5 ml/kg, having first taken a blood specimen for laboratory glucose estimation and for further tests that may be needed later to identify the cause of hypoglycaemia.

First neurological examination

1. Assess Coma Score.
2. Look for signs of impending herniation (see above).

Rapid general physical assessment

Look for evidence of a purpuric rash, injury, enlarged liver, or underlying condition, e.g. presence of ventriculo-peritoneal shunt for hydrocephalus.

While the primary assessment and management is proceeding a history should be obtained as this will give vital clues to the underlying pathology.

> **Specific points for history taking:**
>
> - Recent trauma
> - History of epilepsy
> - Poison ingestion
> - Recent general health
> - Known chronic condition (e.g. renal disease, cardiac abnormality, diabetes)
> - Last meal
> - Recent trips abroad

Coma that develops slowly over a period of hours or days is usually due to an infection (meningitis, encephalitis), a metabolic disturbance (e.g. Reye's syndrome), or a mass lesion. Sudden onset suggests an epileptic seizure, poisoning or, more rarely, a vascular event. Previous episodes of coma suggest certain inborn errors of metabolism (e.g. hyperammonaemia), endocrine disease (e.g. diabetes), epilepsy, porphyria, or repeated poisoning (Meadow's syndrome).

"Treat the treatable"

If the child is stable with regard to cardiorespiratory function, at this stage specific conditions may have been identified and should be treated during primary assessment and management, for example:

- Hypoglycaemia.
- Poisoning with opiates (see Chapter 13).
- Diabetes (see Appendix B).
- Meningococcal septicaemia (see Chapter 9).

Additionally, unless meningitis can be excluded by the clear identification of another cause for coma, treatment should be commenced with penicillin and cefotaxime intravenously (see below). Acyclovir should also be commenced as herpes encephalitis has a worse prognosis when treatment is delayed.

Lumbar puncture should not be performed in a child in coma.

Monitor
- Pulse rate and rhythm.
- Respiratory rate and pattern.
- Core temperature.
- Pulse oximetry.
- Blood pressure.
- Fluid balance.
- Coma Score.
- Chest radiograph.

Early investigations
- Glucose.
- Electrolytes.
- Urea.
- Calcium, magnesium, phosphate.
- Full blood count.
- Blood culture.
- Arterial blood gas.

Secondary assessment and management

In the *secondary* phase, and if the situation is stable, a thorough investigation can be undertaken to ascertain the cause of the coma. If the situation remains unstable or is deteriorating, further urgent primary phase assessment and management must be initiated. It is often impossible to be certain of the diagnosis in the first hour. The main immediate aims are therefore to maintain homoeostasis and "treat the treatable".

Initially the child should be assessed for clinical evidence of raised intracranial pressure (ICP). There are very few absolute signs of raised ICP, and these are papilloedema, a bulging fontanelle, and absence of venous pulsation in retinal vessels. All three signs are often absent in acutely raised ICP.

In a previously well, unconscious child (Glasgow Coma Scale ≤ 8) who is *not* in a post-ictal state, the signs in the box are suggestive of raised intracranial pressure:

Signs of raised intracranial pressure

1. Abnormal oculocephalic reflexes; avoid in patients with neck injuries:
   (a) when the head is rotated to the left or right a normal response is for the eyes to move away from the head movement; an abnormal response is no or random movement;
   (b) when the head is flexed, a normal response is deviation of the eyes upward; a loss of this conjugate upward gaze is a sign suggestive of raised ICP.
2. Abnormal posture:
   (a) decorticate (flexed arms, extended legs);
   (b) decerebrate (extended arms, extended legs).
   Posturing may need to be elicited by a painful stimulus.
3. Abnormal pupillary responses – unilateral or bilateral dilatation suggests raised ICP.
4. Abnormal breathing patterns – there are several recognisable breathing pattern abnormalities in raised ICP. However, they are often changeable and may vary from hyperventilation to Cheyne–Stokes breathing to apnoea.
5. Cushing's triad: slow pulse, raised blood pressure, and breathing pattern abnormalities are a late sign of raised ICP.

If raised intracranial pressure is suspected consult with a paediatric neurologist/neurosurgeon and the following treatment can be commenced:

- Raise head end of patient trolley to 30° with horizontal. Ensure a neutral position of the neck.
- Paralyse, intubate, and hyperventilate to $P\text{CO}_2$ of 3·46–3·72 kPa (26–28 mmHg).
- Give mannitol 0·25–0·5 g/kg intravenously. Mannitol should not be used if the patient is anuric. If in doubt give frusemide 1 mg/kg intravenously first. The child should be catheterised as the bladder may become very full. There is sometimes a "rebound" increase in ICP 2–3 hours after giving mannitol.

Further neurological examination

This should reassess the earlier findings, help localise the site of neurological dysfunction, and provide a reference for further examinations.

1. Eye examination:
   (a) pupil size and reactivity (see box);
   (b) fundal changes – haemorrhage and papilloedema;
   (c) eye deviation – conjugate deviation:
      (i) in cerebral lesions the eyes deviate towards a destructive lesion and away from an irritative lesion;
      (ii) in brain-stem lesions, the eyes deviate away from a destructive lesion;
   (d) reflex ocular movements.
      The oculocephalic reflexes should be reassessed. In the patient with a neck injury, the oculovestibular reflexes may be used. The eyes will deviate towards an ear irrigated with ice cold water in a patient with an intact brain stem.
2. Reassess posture and tone – look for lateralisation.
3. Assess deep tendon reflexes and plantar responses.
4. Reassess Coma Score.

Summary of pupillary changes

Pupil size and reactivity	Cause
Small reactive pupils	Metabolic disorders
	Medullary lesion
Pinpoint fixed pupils	Metabolic disorders
	Opiate/barbiturate/organophosphate ingestions
Fixed mid-size pupils	Mid-brain lesion
Fixed dilated pupils	Hypothermia
	Severe hypoxia
	Barbiturates (late sign)
	During and post-seizure
	Anticholinergic drugs
	Irreversible brain damage
Unilateral dilated pupil	Rapidly expanding ipsilateral lesion, e.g. subdural haematoma
	Tentorial herniation
	Third nerve nucleus lesion
	Epileptic seizures

General physical examination

The physical examination must be thorough and complete. Specific points to include are the following:

1. Skin: rash, haemorrhage, trauma, evidence of neurocutaneous syndromes.
2. Scalp: evidence of trauma.
3. Ears and nose:
   (a) bloody or clear discharge;
   (b) evidence of otitis media.
4. Neck: tenderness or rigidity or tilt.
5. Odour: metabolic disorders and poisoning.
6. Abdomen: enlarged liver.

Further·investigations that may be required include the following:

- Toxicology screen.
- Liver enzymes.
- Blood ammonia.
- Urinary metabolic screen.
- Chest radiograph.
- CT scan.
- Blood smears for parasites.

Lumbar puncture is contraindicated until after neurological consultation.

TRANSFER

Children who remain very ill and those in whom the cause of coma is as yet unidentified will require referral to a paediatric neurologist and may need transfer to a paediatric intensive care unit.

Patients may need paralysis, intubation, and ventilation for safe transfer (see Chapter 24). In such patients neurological assessment cannot be continued, and there should therefore be clear documentation of neurological signs before paralysis is commenced. Similarly, convulsions may be cryptic in a paralysed patient (although raised pulse or blood pressure may suggest ictal activity). Convulsions still increase cerebral metabolic activity even when cryptic. Paralysis should be lightened intermittently to allow assessment of patients at risk of convulsions.

SOME SPECIFIC CONDITIONS

Bacterial meningitis

After the neonatal period, the organisms that cause bacterial meningitis are, in order of frequency, *Haemophilus influenzae*, *Neisseria meningitides* (meningococci), and *Streptococcus pneumoniae*. The overall incidence of bacterial meningitis has remained unchanged for several years at a rate of about 18 per 100 000 children per year. There is still a mortality rate of more than 5% and a similar rate of permanent serious neurological sequelae. Widespread Hib vaccination should reduce the incidence of *Haemophilus influenzae* infection.

Diagnosis of bacterial meningitis
In the under 3-year-old child Bacterial meningitis is the most common and yet the most difficult to diagnose in its early stages in this age group. The classic signs of neck rigidity, photophobia, headache, and vomiting are often absent. A bulging fontanelle is a sign of advanced meningitis in an infant, but even this serious and late sign will be masked if the baby is dehydrated from fever and vomiting. Almost all children with meningitis have some degree of raised intracranial pressure, so that, in fact, the signs and symptoms of meningitis are primarily those of raised intracranial pressure. The following are signs of possible meningitis in infants and young children:

- Coma.
- Drowsiness (often shown by lack of eye contact with parents or doctor).
- Irritability that cannot be easily soothed by parent.
- Poor feeding.
- Unexplained pyrexia.

- Convulsions with or without fever.
- Apnoeic or cyanotic attacks.
- Purpuric rash.

Older children of 4 years and over These children are more likely to have the classic signs of headache, vomiting, pyrexia, neck stiffness, and photophobia. Some present with coma or convulsions. In all unwell children, and children with an unexplained pyrexia, a careful search should be made for neck stiffness and for a purpuric rash. The finding of such a rash in an ill child is almost pathognomic of meningococcal infection for which immediate treatment is required (see Chapter 9).

Lumbar puncture

The purpose of a lumbar puncture is to confirm the diagnosis of meningitis and to identify the organism and its antibiotic sensitivity. There is a risk of coning and death if a lumbar puncture is performed in a child with significantly raised intracranial pressure. Normal fundi are quite consistent with acutely, severely raised intracranial pressure. The relative contraindications to a lumbar puncture are shown in the box.

Relative contraindications to lumbar puncture

- Prolonged or focal seizures
- Focal neurological signs, e.g. asymmetry of limb movement and reflexes, ocular palsies
- A widespread purpuric rash in an ill child – in this case intravenous penicillin and cefotaxime should be given immediately after a blood culture
- Glasgow Coma Scale – score of less than 13
- Pupillary dilatation
- Impaired oculocephalic reflexes (doll's eye reflexes)
- Abnormal posture or movement – decerebrate or decorticate posturing or cycling movements of the limbs
- Inappropriately low pulse, elevated blood pressure, and irregular respirations (i.e. signs of impending brain herniation)
- Coagulation disorder
- Papilloedema
- Hypertension

Treatment

If the child is very seriously ill with a purpuric rash, focal neurological signs, or a decreased conscious level, then antibiotic and supportive treatment should be started after blood for culture and throat swab have been taken. A lumbar puncture should not be done as it may precipitate coning. An initial dose of intravenous penicillin 50 mg/kg (up to a maximum of 2 g) and cefotaxime 50 mg/kg should be given. The antibiotics should be given slowly over 10–15 minutes. If the child is deteriorating neurologically then mannitol 0·5 g/kg can be given and the child be nursed in the 30° head-up position. Consideration should be given to ventilation and the child should be transferred to intensive care. There is now evidence that dexamethasone (0·15 mg/kg) given intravenously before or at the same time as the initial antibiotic improves outcome in some cases.

Reye's syndrome

This relatively uncommon condition is characterised by a rapidly progressive encephalopathy with hypoglycaemia and fatty changes in the liver. Some cases follow varicella or influenza infection. These children appear to improve from their first illness and then become unwell again with profuse vomiting and progressive drowsiness. Other children do not appear to have a prodromal illness. An alleged association with aspirin has led to the banning of aspirin for general use in children less than 12 years of age.

Children with Reye's syndrome present with vomiting, drowsiness, convulsions, or coma. The liver is palpably enlarged and firm. The blood sugar is very low and liver enzymes and serum ammonia are raised.

Although the condition is relatively uncommon, a high index of suspicion should be maintained for Reye's syndrome in patients presenting with profuse vomiting, neurological changes, or hypoglycaemia. Patients can make a good recovery if the disease is recognised early and vigorous treatment instituted rapidly.

The mainstays of treatment are management of the hypoglycaemia and the raised intracranial pressure. For the latter, the patient needs to be transferred to a paediatric intensive care unit for intracranial pressure monitoring and treatment of raised intracranial pressure. While awaiting transfer, the patient should be kept in a head-up position and fluids restricted. If there is continuing deterioration, intubation and ventilation should be instituted and intravenous mannitol given.

13

Poisoning

EPIDEMIOLOGY

Suspected poisoning in children results in about 40 000 attendances at accident and emergency departments each year in England and Wales. Around half of these children are admitted to hospital for treatment or observation. Precise data on hospital admissions for poisonings are altered by the fact that many accident and emergency departments and paediatric wards have special areas where children who have taken a substance of low toxicity can be observed for a few hours without being formally admitted.

Deaths from ingested poisons are uncommon, and are due to drugs (especially tricyclic antidepressants), household products, and rarely plants. As can be seen from Table 13.1, many more children die each year from inhalation of carbon monoxide and other gases in household fires, than die from accidental poisoning by drugs.

Table 13.1. Deaths in children (ages 1–14) from poisons

Cause of death	1987	Deaths in 1988	1989
From poisoning by drugs, medicaments, and biological substances	7	16	16
From toxic effects of carbon monoxide	38	36	36
From toxic effect of other gases, fumes, or vapours	38	56	56

Office of Population Censuses and Surveys, HMSO.

There has been a steady decline in the number of childhood deaths from poisonings. The selective introduction of child-resistant containers in 1976, together with other measures, has reduced the number of poisonings and hospital attendances. In the case of salicylate poisoning the introduction of child-resistant containers saw an 85% fall in hospital admissions from 1975 to 1978. It should, however, be remembered that 20% of children under the age of 5 years are capable of opening child-resistant containers.

AETIOLOGY

Accidental poisoning

This is usually a problem of the young child or toddler, with a mean age of presentation of $2\frac{1}{2}$ years. Accidental poisoning usually occurs when the child is unsupervised, and there is an increased incidence in poisoning following recent disruption in households such as a new baby, moving house, or where there is maternal depression.

Intentional overdose

Suicide or parasuicide attempts are usually made by girls in their teens. These children or adolescents should be admitted to hospital and undergo full psychiatric and social assessment. The assessment of many adolescent self-harm patients in the accident and emergency department has been found to be unsatisfactory. It has been recommended that all children should be promptly assessed as inpatients by a member of a child psychiatry team.

Drug abuse

Alcohol and solvent abuse are the most common forms of drug abuse in children in the UK.

Iatrogenic

The most common drug is diphenoxylate with atropine. This combination is toxic to some children at therapeutic doses. The most frequently fatal drug is digoxin.

Deliberate poisoning

Rarely, symptoms are induced in children by adults via the administration of drugs. A history of poisoning will often not be given at presentation.

PRESENTATION

History

What?
Ask accompanying adults to bring to hospital the container with its remaining contents, or specimen berries or plants that have been eaten. Take a careful note of trade names and all constituents of anything that might have been ingested, as your local poisons unit will need all the details in order to advise you.

How much?
Assume the worst, so if ten tablets are missing assume the child has eaten them all.

When?
This is important for the timing of blood levels, and deciding on appropriate stomach-emptying procedures.

Why?

Was the poisoning accidental, and if so how could it have been avoided? Remember non-accidental injury.

Absent history?

Always suspect poisoning in any child with signs that cannot otherwise be explained, especially the following:

- Drowsiness or coma.
- Convulsions.
- Tachypnoea.
- Tachycardia or flushing.
- Cardiac arrhythmia or hypotension.
- Unusual behaviour.
- Pupillary abnormalities.

Various drugs cause specific signs when taken in overdose and these are summarised in Table 13.2.

Table 13.2. Signs of specific poisonings

Pinpoint pupils	Opiates, organophosphates
Dilated pupils	Atropine, tricyclics
Drowsiness	Alcohol, sedatives, opiates, hypnotics, diphenoxylate/atropine, aspirin, tricyclics
Confusion, ataxia, excitability	Alcohol, tricyclics, antihistamines, salbutamol, solvent abuse
Convulsions	Alcohol, tricyclics, theophylline, lithium
Dystonic reactions	Phenothiazines (e.g. prochlorperazine), metoclopramide
Cardiac arrhythmias	Tricyclics, theophylline, salbutamol, digoxin, potassium
Tachypnoea	Salicylates
Hypotension	Sedatives, hypnotics, iron
Hypertension with tachycardia	Sympathomimetics
Haematemesis	Iron, salicylates

Full and careful examination of the child should follow the ABCD protocol with resuscitative measures as appropriate (see below); remember to record vital signs such as respiratory and pulse rate, blood pressure, and conscious level.

GENERAL MANAGEMENT OF THE SYMPTOMATIC POISONED CHILD

Airway

If the conscious level is depressed and the gag reflex is lost, the airway must be protected by passing an endotracheal tube, unless there is the possibility of rapidly reversing poisoning such as with naloxone for an opiate overdose. The anaesthetist should use a cuffed tube in the older child to protect the airway, particularly if gastric lavage is performed.

Breathing

Check that the respiratory rate and depth are adequate. A pulse oximeter is helpful in assessing adequate tissue oxygenation, and an arterial blood gas estimation should be taken if the child is unconscious or there is concern about adequacy of respiration. If necessary the child should be ventilated.

Circulation

Gain intravenous access. If there is hypotension, fluid resuscitation with an initial bolus of 20 ml/kg of crystalloid should be given. Monitor ECG trace. (See Chapter 10 for dysrhythmia management.)

Disability

Assess pupil size and response to light and level of consciousness using the AVPU system before going on to the full neurological assessment later. Control convulsions (see Chapter 11).

Monitor

- ECG.
- Blood pressure (use appropriate size cuff).
- Pulse oximetry.
- Core temperature.

Estimate blood glucose, urea and electrolytes, and blood gases where indicated.

Consider

- Specific antidotes: opiates, paracetamol, iron, carbon monoxide, cyanide, cholinesterase inhibitors, digoxin, ethylene glycol.
- Assay for paracetamol, salicylate, theophylline, or iron if suspected. (Sample size need not be large; consider the analysis of urine, gastric aspirate, or vomitus.)
- Chest radiograph (consider the risk of aspiration).

Elimination of the poison

Always seek advice from your local Poisons Information Service about the toxicity of potential poisons that the child has taken, unless it is a drug the effects of which are familiar to you. Many children do not need stomach evacuation as they have not taken anything dangerous.

Because of conflicting evidence from clinical studies on poisoned patients, and those utilising adult volunteers, there is continuing controversy over the best way to empty the stomach of ingested poisons. Whether this is done by gastric lavage or by emesis induced with ipecac, less than half of the poison is retrieved.

Emesis

This may be induced with 15 ml ipecac (paediatric) given with a drink and repeated after 30 minutes if necessary. Ninety-five per cent of children will vomit following this treatment, but its active alkaloids can be sedative, and ipecac should never be given to children who are not fully conscious and alert. It should never be given when corrosives have been taken.

Gastric lavage

This is obviously distressing and difficult to perform in children, and is not without risk. Because of limitations of size in children, tablets and capsules are often too large to pass through the entry hole or the tube itself in gastric lavage. It is unlikely to be of any value if more than 4 hours have elapsed since ingestion, unless the drug is aspirin, an antiemetic, or a tricyclic antidepressant. If the child is unconscious without a gag reflex, it is mandatory that the child is first endotracheally intubated to protect the airway and control respiration if necessary.

Summary

If the child is suspected of having ingested a potentially toxic substance within 4 hours, or aspirin, antiemetic, tricyclic antidepressants, or opiates within 12 hours, and if the child is fully conscious and alert, then emesis should be induced with ipecac providing that the poison is not corrosive.

Gastric lavage is indicated in the following situations:

- After endotracheal intubation in an unconscious poisoned child (seek anaesthetic help).
- In patients who cannot be persuaded to take ipecac or who have not vomited after two doses.
- In paraquat poisoning, when fuller's earth can be introduced after the washout.
- In children who have taken large doses of insoluble aspirin or iron tablets in an attempt to break up concretions of the stomach, and to administer desferrioxamine in the case of iron poisoning.

Reducing absorption of poisons

Activated charcoal

This is thought to act by combining with drugs to prevent their intestinal absorption. It is black and unpalatable, and therefore it is extremely difficult to encourage a child to drink it. To be maximally effective, a charcoal:drug ratio of 10:1 is necessary. Although effective this treatment is sometimes impracticable in children.

Activated charcoal is, however, particularly effective for treatment of poisoning with tricyclic antidepressants, theophylline (repeated doses every 4 hours), digoxin, and barbiturates, and is best introduced into the stomach via the gastric lavage tube once the stomach has been emptied. It cannot be used with ipecac.

SPECIFIC POISONS

In most poisoning cases, the usual ABC approach will stabilise the patient and allow detailed up-to-the-minute advice to be sought from the Poisons Centre. The following are some of the more common drugs for which very urgent specific treatment may be required.

Iron

The child with iron poisoning presents in shock which may be due to gut haemorrhage. Intubation, ventilation, and circulatory support are necessary in the severely affected child. Gastric lavage can be performed once the airway is secured. Specific therapy is to infuse desferrioxamine 15 mg/kg/h. At this infusion rate hypotension should not be a problem.

Tricyclic antidepressant

Tricyclic antidepressant poisoning causes anticholinergic effects (tachycardia, dilated pupils, convulsions) and cardiac effects (conduction delay, any arrhythmia). Convulsions should be treated as described in Chapter 11 and arrhythmias as in Chapter 10 (but see later).

Additionally, alkalinisation up to an arterial pH of 7·5 has been shown to reduce the toxic effects on the heart. This can be achieved by hyperventilation ($P\text{co}_2$ no lower than 3·33 kPa (25 mmHg)) and by infusing sodium bicarbonate (1 mmol/kg). Phenytoin enhances conduction and is the drug of choice for arrhythmias (18 mg/kg over 20–30 min). Lignocaine may be helpful. Quinidine, procainamide, and disopyramide are contraindicated.

Opiates and methadone

Following stabilisation of airway, breathing, and circulation, the specific antidote is naloxone. An initial bolus dose of 100 µg/kg up to a maximum of 2 mg should be given. Naloxone has a short half-life and further boluses, or an infusion of 10–20 µg/kg/min or more, may be required.

Telephone numbers of National Poisons Centres

London	071-955 5095 or 071-635 9191
Edinburgh	031-229 2477
Cardiff	0222-709 901
Leeds	0532-430 715
Birmingham	021-554 3801
Newcastle	091-232 5131
Belfast	0232-240 503
Dublin	0001-379 964

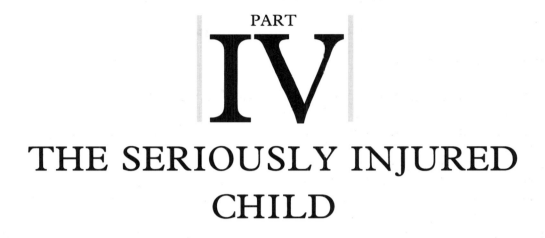

PART

IV

THE SERIOUSLY INJURED CHILD

14

Initial assessment and management

This chapter sets out a structured approach to the initial assessment and management of the seriously injured child. Children and adults are affected quite differently by major injuries – physically, physiologically, and psychologically. A young child cannot describe pain, or even localise symptoms. The more frightened children become, the "younger" they behave, and the less they can contribute to management. All symptoms may be denied vehemently.

Although traumatised children have a number of unique problems, this in no way affects the validity of a structured approach. By following the principles outlined, problems will be identified and treated in order of priority. It should be emphasised from the start that, although assessment and management are discussed separately, this is purely to allow things to be shown clearly. When dealing with an injured child it is essential that appropriate resuscitative measures are taken as soon as a problem is found.

The form of the structured approach is shown in the box.

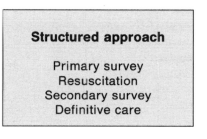

Structured approach

Primary survey
Resuscitation
Secondary survey
Definitive care

PRIMARY SURVEY

During the primary survey life-threatening conditions are identified. Assessment follows the familiar ABC pattern with significant additions:

A Airway and cervical spine control
B Breathing
C Circulation and haemorrhage control
D Disability
E Exposure

Airway and cervical spine

Airway assessment following trauma should follow the

LOOK
LISTEN
FEEL

technique discussed in Chapters 4 and 5.

A cervical spine injury should be assumed to be present until adequate investigation and examination exclude it.

Breathing

Once the airway has been secured and the cervical spine controlled, breathing should be assessed. As discussed in earlier chapters the adequacy of breathing is gained from three sets of observations – the work of breathing, the effectiveness of breathing, and the effects of inadequate respiration on other organ systems. These are summarised in the box.

Assessment of the adequacy of breathing

The work of breathing
  Recession
  Respiratory rate
  Inspiratory or expiratory noises
  Grunting
  Accessory muscle use
  Flare of the alae nasi
Effectiveness of breathing
  Breath sounds
  Chest expansion
  Abdominal excursion
Effects of inadequate respiration
  Heart rate
  Skin colour
  Mental status

The normal resting respiratory rate changes with age. These changes are summarised in Table 14.2.

Circulation

Circulatory assessment in the primary survey consists of the rapid assessment of heart rate, systolic blood pressure, capillary refill time, skin colour and temperature, respiratory rate, and mental status. Using these measures an approximate estimate of the percentage of blood loss can be made as shown in Table 14.1.

Table 14.1. Recognition of stages of shock

Sign	Assessment of percentage blood loss		
	<25	25–40	>40
Heart rate	Tachycardia+	Tachycardia++	Tachycardia/ bradycardia
Systolic BP	Normal	Normal or falling	Falling
Pulse volume	Normal/reduced	Reduced+	Reduced++
Capillary refill time (Normal <2 s)	Normal/increased	Increased+	Increased++
Skin	Cool, pale	Cold, mottled	Cold Pale
Respiratory rate	Tachypnoea+	Tachypnoea++	Sighing respiration
Mental state	Mild agitation	Lethargic Uncooperative	Reacts only to pain

Resting heart rate, blood pressure, and respiratory rate vary with age, and circulatory assessment of a child must take this variation into account. The normal values are shown in Table 14.2.

Table 14.2. Vital signs: approximate range of normal

Age (years)	Respiratory rate (breaths/min)	Systolic BP (mmHg)	Pulse (beats/min)
<1	30–40	70–90	110–160
2–5	25–30	80–100	95–140
5–12	20–25	90–110	80–120
>12	15–20	100–120	60–100

Disability

The assessment of disability during the primary survey consists of a brief neurological examination to determine conscious level, and assessment of pupil size and reactivity. Conscious level determination is kept as simple as possible – and requires only that the child is put into one of the four following categories:

A   Alert
V   Responds to Voice
P   Responds to Pain
U   Unresponsive

Exposure

In order to assess a seriously injured child fully, it is necessary to take his or her clothes off. Children become cold very quickly, and may be acutely embarrassed when undressed in front of strangers. Although exposure is necessary the time taken for it should be minimised, and a blanket provided at all other times.

131

RESUSCITATION

Life-threatening problems should be treated as they are identified during the primary survey.

Airway and cervical spine

Airway

The airway may be compromised by extrinsic material (blood, vomit, or a foreign body), by the tongue, or by injury to the face, mouth, or upper airway. Whatever the cause, airway management should follow the sequence described in Chapters 4 and 5. This is summarised in the box.

Airway management sequence

- Jaw thrust
- Suction/removal of foreign body
- Oral/pharyngeal airways
- Endotracheal intubation
- Surgical airway

Head tilt/chin lift is not recommended following trauma, because cervical spine injuries may be exacerbated.

Cervical spine

The cervical spine should be presumed to be damaged until proved intact, especially if there is obvious injury above the clavicle. Children can have significant spinal cord injury without radiographic abnormality (with devastating consequences if ignored). Even if normal radiographs are obtained the cervical spine must be protected in any patient where there is a high index of suspicion. If the child is unconscious or cooperative, his or her head and neck should be immobilised initially by in-line manual stabilisation, and then using a semi-rigid collar, sandbags, and tape. Uncooperative or combative patients should simply have a hard collar applied, because too rigid immobilisation of the head in such cases may increase neck movement as struggling occurs. Only when radiographs are normal, *and* the neurological examination has been demonstrated to be completely normal, should immobilising manoeuvres be discontinued.

Breathing

If breathing is inadequate, ventilation must be commenced. Initially bag–mask ventilation should be performed. Generally speaking, a child who requires bag–mask ventilation initially following trauma will subsequently require intubation to control the airway. Following intubation, mechanical ventilation can be commenced.

The indications for intubation and mechanical ventilation are summarised in the box.

Indications for intubation and ventilation

- Inadequate oxygenation via bag-and-mask technique
- Prolonged ventilation required
- Therapeutic hyperventilation required
- Flail chest
- Inhalational burn injury
- Shock

If breath sounds are unequal then pneumothorax, misplaced endotracheal tube, or blocked main bronchus should be considered, and appropriate measures should be taken.

Circulation

All seriously injured children require urgent establishment of vascular access. Two relatively large intravenous cannulae are mandatory. The percutaneous approach to peripheral veins is the preferred route, but, if this fails, other routes should be used. The external jugular veins and femoral veins can be cannulated, and a cut-down onto the cephalic vein at the elbow or long saphenous at the ankle should be considered. Intraosseous infusion may be used, and will usually prove quicker and easier than the more specialised techniques mentioned above. Vascular access techniques are discussed in detail in Chapter 22.

Central venous cannulation is particularly hazardous in children, and should not be attempted by the inexperienced. If a central venous line is inserted, its main use is for monitoring central venous pressure.

Fluid therapy should be commenced as a bolus using 20 ml/kg of crystalloid (e.g. normal (physiological) saline) or colloid (e.g. 4·5% human albumin solution). The response should be assessed. If there is no change, a further bolus of fluid is given. If there is still no improvement, the next bolus should be of whole blood or packed cells, and a surgical opinion should be sought urgently – this is summarised in Figure 14.1.

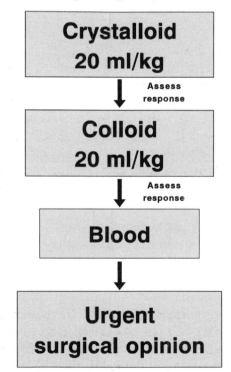

Figure 14.1. Fluids in hypovolaemic shock after trauma

Cross-matching of blood takes time, and clinical urgency may dictate that type-specific or O-negative blood must be given. The times necessary to obtain blood are shown in Table 14.3.

Table 14.3. Cross-match times

Blood type	Cross-match	Time (minutes)
O negative	Nil	0
Type specific	ABO	10–15
Full cross-match	Full	45–60

Other procedures carried out during resuscitation

History taking

History should be sought from the child, ambulance personnel, relatives, and witnesses of the accident. Ambulance staff should be able to provide a great deal of information, including details of the accident site and of pre-hospital care that was administered. Relatives should be able to give the child's past medical history and allergies, and provide details of the time of the last meal.

The mechanism of injury is useful in assessment. The information in Table 14.4 should be obtained if possible.

Table 14.4. Relevant history of injury mechanism

Road accident	Other
Car occupant/cyclist/pedestrian	Nature of accident
Position in vehicle	Objects involved
Restraints worn	Height of fall
Head protection	Landing surface
Thrown from vehicle	Environmental
Speed of impact	Temperature
Damage to the vehicle	Contamination
Other victims' injuries	

Blood tests

At the same time that intravenous access is obtained, blood should be taken for baseline haematology, baseline biochemistry, and cross-matching.

Radiographs

All seriously injured children must have radiographs of the *lateral cervical spine*, *chest*, and *pelvis*. Other radiographs are taken as dictated by clinical examination.

Urinary catheterisation

Catheterisation of a child should only be performed if the child cannot pass urine spontaneously, or if continuous accurate output measurement is required. The route (urethral or suprapubic) will depend on factors related to signs of urethral, bladder, or intra-abdominal injury. If a boy requires urethral catheterisation, urethral damage must be excluded first. The smallest Silastic catheter should be used in order to reduce the risk of subsequent urethral stricture formation. Urine should be sent for microscopy.

Nasogastric tube placement

Acute gastric dilatation is common in children and the stomach should be decompressed. If there is suspicion of base of skull fracture the tube should be passed orally.

Analgesia

Analgesia should be considered at this stage and administered unless there is very good reason for not doing so. Morphine is the drug of choice and should be given intravenously in a dose of 0·1 mg/kg. There is no place for the administration of intramuscular analgesia in trauma. Entonox (a 50/50 mix of O_2/N_2O) should be considered, but is contraindicated if there is a possibility of pneumothorax or base of skull fractures.

SECONDARY SURVEY

When the primary survey has been completed and resuscitation has stabilised the patient, the secondary survey can be started. If simple resuscitative measures do not stabilise the child, then operative intervention may be necessary before a formal secondary survey is undertaken. Whenever it is performed, it should identify all the injuries present in an anatomical and methodical way, and entails a thorough clinical examination, and relevant investigations.

Throughout this stage of management, the vital signs and neurological status should be continually reassessed, and any deterioration should lead to an immediate return to the primary survey.

Head

Clinical examination
- Inspect for bruising, haemorrhage, deformity, and CSF leak.
- Palpate for lacerations, bruising, and skull depressions.
- Perform otoscopy and ophthalmoscopy.
- Perform a mini-neurological examination:
    pupillary reflexes;
    Glasgow Coma Scale assessment (see Chapter 17);
    motor function – reflexes, tone, power.

Investigations (as indicated)
- Skull radiographs.
- CT brain scan.

Face

Clinical examination
- Inspect for bruising, lacerations, and deformity.
- Inspect the mouth inside and out.
- Palpate the bones for deformity.
- Palpate the teeth for looseness.

Investigations (as indicated)
  Facial radiographs.

Neck

Clinical examination

Care should be taken not to move the cervical spine during this assessment. If the semi-rigid collar is removed, an assistant should maintain in-line cervical stabilisation throughout.

- Inspect the front and back of the neck for bruising and swelling.
- Palpate the cervical spine for tenderness, bruising, swelling, and deformity.
- Palpate for surgical emphysema.

Investigations (as indicated)
Further cervical spine radiographs:

- Anteroposterior view.
- Odontoid view.
- Oblique view.
- CT scan.

Flexion and extension views should *not* be obtained without specialist advice.

Chest

Clinical examination
- Inspect for bruising, lacerations, deformity, and movement.
- Inspect neck veins.
- Feel for tracheal deviation.
- Feel for tenderness, crepitus, and paradoxical movement.
- Percuss.
- Listen for breath sounds and added sounds.
- Listen for heart sounds.

Investigations (as indicated)
- ECG.
- Further chest radiographs.
- Special radiographs as indicated (e.g. tomogram, aortogram).
- CT scan.

Abdomen

Clinical examination
- Observe for movement.
- Inspect for bruising, lacerations, and swelling.
- Palpate for tenderness, rigidity, and masses.
- Auscultate for bowel sounds.

Internal examinations should be performed by the responsible surgeon so as to avoid unnecessary repetition of upsetting procedures.

Investigations (as indicated)
- Ultrasound.
- CT scan.

- Diagnostic peritoneal lavage.
- Intravenous urogram (pyelogram).

Pelvis

Clinical examination
- Inspect for bruising, lacerations, and deformity.
- Inspect the perineum.
- Inspect the external urethral meatus for blood.
- Press over the anterior iliac crest for elicited tenderness and abnormal mobility.

Investigations (as indicated)
- Bladder ultrasound.
- Retrograde urethrography.

Spine

Clinical examination

**Proper spinal examination can only be carried out after the child
has been log-rolled (see Chapter 23).**

- Observe for swelling and bruising.
- Palpate for tenderness, bruising, swelling, and deformity.
- Assess motor and sensory function.

Investigations (as indicated)
- Radiographs.
- CT scans.

Extremities

Clinical examination
- Observe for bruising, swelling, and deformity.
- Palpate for tenderness; crepitus and abnormal movement may be found (do not elicit deliberately as these are painful).
- Assess peripheral circulation – pulses and capillary return.
- Assess peripheral sensation – to touch and pin-prick.

Investigations (as indicated)
- Radiographs.
- Angiograms.

CONTINUED MONITORING

Pulse, blood pressure, respiratory rate, pupil size and reactivity, and Glasgow Coma Score should be measured and charted frequently (at least every 15 minutes). Urinary output must be recorded hourly. Oxygen saturation and end-tidal CO_2 (in the ventilated child) provide useful additional information, and should be measured if possible.

Any deterioration should lead to immediate reassessment of the airway, breathing, and circulation, and appropriate resuscitative measures should be commenced.

DEFINITIVE CARE

Definitive care is the final part of the structured approach to trauma, and is often carried out by teams other than that which initially received the patient. Good note-taking and appropriate referral are essential if time is not to be lost. If definitive care is to be undertaken in a specialist centre then secondary transfer may be necessary at this stage.

Note-taking

The structured approach discussed in this chapter can provide a framework for the writing of notes. It is recommended that these should be set out as shown in Figure 14.2.

```
Primary survey
    A
    B
    C
    D
    E

Resuscitation
    A
    B
    C

Secondary survey
    Head
    Face
    Neck
    Chest
    Abdomen
    Pelvis
    Spine
    Extremities
        Upper
        Lower
```

Figure 14.2. Template for note-taking

Referral

Many teams may be involved in the definitive care of a seriously injured child. It is essential that referrals are made appropriately, clearly, and early. Guidance about which children to refer to which teams is given in subsequent chapters.

Transfer

Injured children may require transfer either within the hospital or to another centre. In either case thorough preparation of equipment, patient, and documentation is essential. Secondary transfer should not be undertaken until all life-threatening problems have been addressed, and the child is stable. Transport of children is discussed in more detail in Chapter 24.

SUMMARY

The structured approach to initial assessment and management, discussed here, allows the professional to care for the seriously injured child in a logical, efficacious fashion.

Assessment of vital functions (airway, breathing, and circulation) is carried out first; resuscitation for any problems found is instituted immediately:

- Primary survey.
- Resuscitation.

A complete head-to-toe examination is then carried out, and finally referral to teams responsible for definitive care is made:

- Secondary survey.
- Definitive care.

15

Chest trauma

Following the establishment of a secure airway, the next most important consideration in the resuscitation of a child is the assessment of breathing. The child who has suffered multiple injuries may well have significant intrathoracic trauma that severely compromises respiration, and requires immediate treatment.

Substantial amounts of kinetic energy may be transferred through a child's chest wall with little or no external sign of injury. Furthermore, children have very elastic ribs which rarely fracture; thus a normal chest radiograph does not exclude major thoracic visceral disruption.

Thoracic injuries must be considered in all children who suffer major trauma. Some may be life threatening and require immediate therapy during the primary survey and resuscitation, whereas others may be discovered during the secondary survey. *The vast majority can be managed in the first hour by any competent doctor*. Practical procedures are described in detail in Chapter 23.

INJURIES POSING AN IMMEDIATE THREAT TO LIFE

Tension pneumothorax

This is a life-threatening emergency. Air accumulates under pressure in the pleural space; this, in turn, pushes the mediastinum across the chest and kinks the great vessels in the mediastinum. This then compromises venous return to the heart and therefore cardiac output is reduced. The diagnosis is a clinical one. A radiograph that shows a tension pneumothorax should never have been taken.

Signs
- The child will be hypoxic and may be shocked.
- There will be decreased air entry and hyperresonance to percussion on the side of the pneumothorax.
- Distended neck veins may be apparent in thin children.
- Later the trachea will be deviated away from the side of the pneumothorax.

Therapy
- High-flow oxygen should be given through a reservoir mask.
- Immediate needle thoracocentesis should be performed to relieve the tension.
- A chest drain should be inserted urgently to prevent recurrence.

Air may be forced into the pneumothorax by artificial ventilation. Any patient with a pneumothorax will develop a tension pneumothorax if ventilated.

Massive haemopneumothorax

Air and blood accumulate in the pleural space. This results from damage to the lung parenchyma with possible additional damage to pulmonary or chest wall blood vessels. The hemithorax can contain a substantial proportion of a child's blood volume.

Signs
- The child will be hypoxic and in shock.
- There will be decreased chest movement, decreased air entry, and decreased resonance to percussion on the side of the haemopneumothorax.

Treatment
- High-flow oxygen should be given through a reservoir mask.
- Intravenous access should be established and volume replacement commenced.
- A relatively large chest drain should be inserted urgently.

Open pneumothorax

There is a penetrating wound in the chest wall with associated pneumothorax. The wound may be obvious, but it may be on the patient's back, and will not be seen unless actively looked for.

Signs
- Air may be heard sucking and blowing through the wound.
- The other signs of pneumothorax will be present.

Treatment
- High-flow oxygen should be given through a reservoir mask.
- The wound should be occluded (on three sides only in order to allow air to escape otherwise a tension pneumothorax will be created).
- A chest drain should be inserted urgently.

Flail chest

The elasticity of the child's chest wall reduces the incidence of flail chest, on the one hand. On the other, the increased mobility means that children are badly affected by these injuries if they do occur, because the underlying lung injury tends to be worse. Anteroposterior or posteroanterior chest radiographs do not demonstrate rib fractures reliably and should not be relied upon in making the diagnosis.

Signs
- The child will be hypoxic.
- Abnormal chest movement associated with rib crepitus may be seen.
- Flail segments may not be seen on initial examination because reflex splinting of the segment occurs.

Treatment
- High-flow oxygen should be given through a reservoir mask.
- Endotracheal intubation and ventilation should be considered.

142

- Adequate pain relief must be given; this is difficult to achieve in children because intercostal nerve blockade is dangerous in the uncooperative patient, and anaesthetic consultation may be required.

Cardiac tamponade

Cardiac tamponade can occur after both penetrating and blunt injury. The blood that accumulates in the fibrous pericardial sac reduces the volume available for cardiac filling during diastole. As more blood accumulates cardiac output is progressively reduced.

Signs
- The child will be in shock.
- There may be muffled heart sounds.
- There may be distended neck veins; this will not be apparent if significant hypovolaemia coexists.

Treatment
- High-flow oxygen should be given through a reservoir mask.
- Intravenous access should be established, and rapid volume replacement commenced; this temporarily increases filling pressure.
- Emergency needle pericardiocentesis should be performed; removal of a small volume of fluid from within the pericardium can dramatically increase cardiac output.

SERIOUS INJURIES DISCOVERED LATER

Pulmonary contusion

Children have a high incidence of pulmonary contusion because of the mobility of the ribs. There may be no overlying fracture. This injury is usually the result of blunt trauma which ruptures pulmonary capillaries allowing blood to fill the alveoli, causing the child to become hypoxic.

Diagnosis is often by exclusion. "Consolidation" may be seen on chest radiograph, but this investigation may be normal. Treatment consists of the administration of high-flow oxygen, and artificial ventilation if necessary.

Tracheal and bronchial rupture

Frequently lethal, this presents as a pneumo- or haemopneumothorax, possibly with associated subcutaneous emphysema.

Immediate treatment is as described above. Continued significant air leaks after chest drain insertion strongly suggest this diagnosis. Further treatment requires referral to a cardiothoracic surgeon.

Disruption of great vessels

This is usually rapidly fatal. A child with this injury who survives to get to hospital has a tear in a vessel that has tamponaded itself.

The patient may be shocked and peripheral pulses may be poorly palpable. The diagnosis should be suspected if a widened mediastinum is seen on chest radiograph. A radiologist should be called to perform urgent angiography. Definitive treatment is by a cardiothoracic surgeon.

Ruptured diaphragm

This may occur following blunt abdominal trauma, and is more common on the left side.

The child may be hypoxic due to pulmonary compression, and may have signs of hypovolaemia if intra-abdominal visceral injury has occurred. A chest radiograph often reveals abnormalities caused by the presence of abdominal contents. These may be non-specific, or can be diagnostic if bowel shadowing or an abnormal position for the nasogastric tube is present. A cardiothoracic surgical referral should be made.

OTHER INJURIES

Simple pneumothorax

A self-limiting leak of air occurs. This causes partial lung collapse. Signs of hypoxia are rarely apparent. Clinically, decreased chest wall movement, diminished breath sounds, and hyperresonance may be found on the side of the pneumothorax. The diagnosis is usually made radiologically.

A chest drain should be inserted electively. If the patient is to be ventilated chest drain insertion *must* be undertaken urgently. In the ventilated patient a simple pneumothorax becomes a tension pneumothorax.

PRACTICAL PROCEDURES

Needle thoracocentesis, chest drain insertion, and pericardiocentesis are described in Chapter 23.

REFERRAL

Most immediately life-threatening chest injuries can be successfully managed by a competent doctor. However, cardiothoracic consultation may be required as a result of conditions uncovered by chest drainage and for serious injuries discovered during the secondary survey. The major reasons for referral are shown in the box.

Indications for cardiothoracic surgical referral

Continuing massive air leak after chest drain insertion
Continuing haemorrhage after chest drain insertion
Cardiac tamponade
Disruption of the great vessels

Patients who require ventilation as part of the treatment of their chest injury (such as those with significant pulmonary contusion) will need referral to a paediatric intensive care unit.

144

SUMMARY

A clear airway must be established before attending to chest injuries

All patients should receive high-flow oxygen through a reservoir mask

Chest injuries are life threatening but most can be managed successfully by any doctor capable of performing the following techniques:

- Needle thoracocentesis
- Chest drain insertion
- Intubation and ventilation
- Fluid replacement
- Pericardiocentesis

Cardiothoracic surgical referral may be necessary once immediate management of life-threatening conditions has been carried out

16

Abdominal injuries

Blunt trauma causes the majority of abdominal injuries in children. Most occur because of accidents on the roads, although a significant number happen during recreational activities. A high index of suspicion is necessary if some injuries are not to be missed.

The abdominal contents are very susceptible to injury in children for a number of reasons. The abdominal wall is thin and offers relatively little protection. The diaphragm is more horizontal than in adults, causing the liver and spleen to lie lower and more anteriorly. Furthermore the ribs, being very elastic, offer less protection to these organs. Finally, the bladder is intra-abdominal, rather than pelvic, and is therefore more exposed. Respiratory compromise can complicate abdominal injury because diaphragmatic irritation or splinting may occur – reducing the use of the diaphragm during breathing.

HISTORY

A precise history of the mechanism of injury may help in diagnosis. Rapid deceleration, such as experienced during road accidents, causes abdominal compression. The spleen and liver are at risk from such forces, and the duodenum may develop a large haematoma or may rupture at the duodenojejunal flexure. Direct blows, such as those caused by punching or impact with bicycle handlebars, injure underlying organs. Again the liver and spleen, being relatively exposed, are at risk. Finally, straddling injuries can cause perineal injury and may rupture the urethra.

ASSESSMENT OF THE INJURED ABDOMEN

Initial assessment and management must be directed to the care of the airway, breathing, and circulation as discussed in Chapter 14.

Examination

If shock is not amenable to fluid replacement during the primary survey and resuscitation, and no obvious site of haemorrhage exists, then intra-abdominal injury may be the cause of blood loss. The abdomen should be assessed urgently to establish whether early operative intervention is necessary. In other circumstances, the abdominal examination is carried out during the secondary survey.

The abdomen should be inspected for bruising, lacerations, and penetrating wounds. Major intra-abdominal injury can occur without obvious external signs, and visible bruising is therefore highly significant. The external urethral meatus should be examined for blood.

Gentle palpation should be carried out. This will reveal areas of tenderness and rigidity. Care should be taken not to hurt the child because his or her continued cooperation is important during the repeated examinations that form an important part of management.

Rectal and vaginal examinations are mandatory in an adult with multiple injuries. In children every effort should be made to limit internal examination to that performed by the surgeon who is going to operate on that child. Even then it should only be done if the result of the examination will alter the management.

Aids to assessment

Both gastric and urinary bladder drainage may help the assessment by decompressing the abdomen.

Gastric drainage

Air swallowing during crying with consequent acute gastric dilatation is common in children. Early passage of a *gastric tube* of an appropriate size is essential. The tube should be aspirated regularly and left on free drainage at other times. A massively distended stomach can mimic intra-abdominal pathology needing laparotomy, and cause serious diaphragm splintage with consequent respiratory compromise.

Urinary catheterisation

Catheterisation of a child should only be performed if the child cannot pass urine spontaneously, or if continuous accurate output measurement is required. The route (urethral or suprapubic) will depend on factors related to signs of urethral, bladder, or intra-abdominal injury. If a boy requires urethral catheterisation, urethral damage must be excluded first. The catheter should be Silastic and as small as possible in order to reduce the risk of subsequent urethral stricture formation.

Investigations

Blood tests

Intravenous access will have already been secured during the primary survey and resuscitation, and at that time blood will have been drawn for baseline blood counts, urea and electrolytes, and cross-matching. An amylase estimation should be requested and can usually be performed on the sample sent for urea and electrolytes. Arterial blood gases should be sent if indicated. Repeated monitoring of blood parameters may be appropriate in some patients.

Radiographs Views of the lateral cervical spine, chest, and pelvis will have been obtained during the course of the primary survey. Neither a normal chest radiograph nor a normal pelvic radiograph excludes abdominal injury. A plain abdominal radiograph may be helpful to look for the position of the gastric tube, distribution of abdominal gas, presence of free gas, and soft tissue swellings including a full bladder.

Renal injury may need investigation by intravenous urography. Blood at the external urethral meatus will require investigation using retrograde urethrography.

Computed tomography A CT scan of the abdomen with intravenous and intragastric contrast is the radiological investigation of choice in children. CT will alert the surgeon to solid organ rupture, free intraperitoneal contrast from a perforated viscus, the presence or absence of two functioning kidneys, and free intraperitoneal contrast from a ruptured bladder.

Ultrasound This may be readily available and give early information on free fluid and lacerations in the liver, spleen, or kidneys.

Diagnostic peritoneal lavage This is rarely used in children, as the presence of intraperitoneal blood per se is not necessarily an indication for laparotomy. Once lavage fluid has been introduced, the peritoneum shows signs of irritation for up to 48 hours, and hence reduces the possibility of accurate repeated assessment. Peritoneal lavage should therefore only be carried out by the surgeon managing the case.

A lavage should be considered positive if the red cell count is over $100\,000/\text{mm}^3$, the white cell count over $500/\text{mm}^3$, or if enteric contents or bacteria are seen. Laboratory analysis gives the best specificity and selectivity for this test. Bedside estimation is dangerously unreliable. This technique is described in Chapter 23.

DEFINITIVE CARE

Non-operative management

Until the early 1980s, both adult and paediatric patients with haemoperitoneum would undergo laparotomy. Damage to the spleen or liver would result in splenectomy or partial hepatectomy respectively. It has since been shown that the haemorrhage is often self-limiting, and many of these operations can therefore be avoided. As well as avoiding the morbidity associated with laparotomy, this approach also reduces the number of children at risk of sepsis following splenectomy.

For non-operative management to be undertaken the following are essential:

- Adequate observation and frequent monitoring.
- Precise fluid management.
- The immediate availability of a surgeon trained to operate on the paediatric abdomen (should this become necessary).

The need for clotting factors as platelets, fresh frozen plasma, or cryoprecipitate must be monitored. Vigorous and early management of coagulopathy is indicated, in order to improve clotting and hence achieve haemostasis.

Indications for operative intervention

All children with penetrating abdominal injuries and those with definite signs of bowel perforation will require urgent laparotomy. Children whose circulation is not stable after replacement of 40 ml/kg of fluid are probably bleeding into the thoracic or abdominal cavities. In the absence of clear thoracic bleeding, urgent laparotomy is necessary.

A non-functioning kidney, as demonstrated on contrast studies, may have suffered a major renal pedicle injury. These require immediate exploration to ascertain whether the kidney can be saved. The warm ischaemia time for a kidney is only 45–60 minutes.

Indications for operative intervention following abdominal injury

Laparotomy
    Penetrating injuries
    Signs of bowel perforation
    Refractory shock
Renal exploration
    Non-functioning kidney

It is essential that the surgeon performing these procedures is competent to deal with paediatric trauma and can perform any reconstructive surgery that may be required.

SUMMARY

- The assessment and management of airway, breathing, and circulation must be carried out first. Abdominal assessment is only carried out at this stage if shock is refractory
- Abdominal assessment consists of careful observation and gentle, repeated palpation. Gastric and urinary drainage aid this assessment
- Abdominal CT scan is the investigation of choice. Diagnostic peritoneal lavage is rarely used in children
- Some children with visceral injury may be managed non-operatively if essential requirements are met. Others will need urgent operative intervention

17

Head trauma

EPIDEMIOLOGY

Head injury is the most common single cause of death in children aged 1–15 years. It accounts for 15% of deaths in this age group, and for 25% of deaths in the 5–15 year age group.

The most common occurrence that causes death from head injury is a road traffic accident. Pedestrian children are the most vulnerable, followed by cyclists, and then passengers in vehicles. Falls are the second most common cause of fatal head injuries. In infancy the most common cause is child abuse.

PATHOPHYSIOLOGY

Brain damage may be from the primary or secondary effects of the injury.

Primary damage

- Cerebral lacerations.
- Cerebral contusions.
- Dural sac tears.
- Diffuse axonal injury.

Secondary damage

This may result from either the direct secondary effects of cerebral injury or from the cerebral consequences of associated injuries and stress:

- Hypoxia from inadequate ventilation caused by loss of respiratory drive.
- Hypoxia from airway obstruction or thoracic injuries.
- Ischaemia from poor cerebral perfusion secondary to raised intracranial pressure.
- Ischaemia secondary to hypotension and blood loss.
- Hypoglycaemia.
- Loss of metabolic homoeostasis.
- Hypothermia.
- Fever.
- Convulsions.

151

Raised intracranial pressure

Once sutures have closed at 12–18 months of age, the child's cranial cavity behaves like an adult's with a fixed volume. Cerebral oedema or haematomas increase the volume of the contents. Initial compensatory mechanisms include diminution of the total volume of cerebrospinal fluid and diminution in the pool of venous blood. When these mechanisms fail, volume increase leads to raised intracranial pressure. This causes an increased pressure gradient for the inflow of arterial blood and a fall in cerebral perfusion pressure.

Cerebral perfusion pressure = Mean arterial pressure − Mean intracranial pressure

Normal cerebral blood flow is 50 ml of blood per 100 g brain tissue per minute. A fall in cerebral perfusion pressure decreases cerebral blood flow. A flow of below 20 ml per 100 g of brain tissue per minute will produce ischaemia; this increases cerebral oedema and hence causes a further rise in intracranial pressure. A cerebral blood flow of below 10 ml/100 g/minute leads to electrical dysfunction of the neurones and loss of intracellular homoeostasis.

A generalised increase of intracranial pressure in the supratentorial compartment initially causes trans-tentorial (uncal), and later causes trans-foraminal (central) herniation (coning), and death. Unilateral increases in intracranial pressure secondary to haematoma formation cause ipsilateral uncal herniation. The third nerve is nipped against the free border of the tentorium, causing ipsilateral pupillary dilatation secondary to loss of parasympathetic constrictor tone to the ciliary muscles.

In childhood, the most common cause of raised intracranial pressure following head injury is cerebral oedema. Children are especially prone to this problem. They may, of course, also have expanding extradural, subdural, or intracerebral haematomas which will require surgical treatment.

Depending on the aetiology of the raised intracranial pressure, treatment is either aimed at preventing it rising further, or removing its cause (by surgical evacuation of haematomas).

There are special considerations in infants with head injuries. Their cranial volume can more easily increase because of unfused sutures. Therefore, large extradural or subdural bleeds may occur before neurological signs or symptoms develop. Such infants may show a significant fall in haemoglobin concentration. Additionally, the infant's vascular scalp may bleed profusely causing shock. In children over 1 year with shock associated with head injury, serious extracranial injury should be sought.

PATIENT TRIAGE

Head injuries vary from the trivial to the fatal. Triage is necessary in order to give more seriously injured patients a higher priority. Factors indicating a potentially serious injury are shown in the box.

Factors indicating a potentially serious injury

- History of substantial trauma such as involvement in a road traffic accident or a fall from a height
- A history of loss of consciousness
- Children who are not fully conscious and responsive
- Any child with obvious neurological signs/symptoms such as headache, convulsions, or limb weakness
- Evidence of penetrating injury

ASSESSMENT

Primary survey

The first priority is to assess and stabilise the airway, breathing, and circulation as discussed in Chapter 14. Head injury may be associated with cervical spine injury, and neck immobilisation must be achieved as previously described.

Pupil size and reactivity should be examined, and a rapid assessment of conscious level should be made. The latter consists of placing the child into one of four categories as shown.

A	**Alert**
V	Responds to **Voice**
P	Responds to **Pain**
U	**Unresponsive**

The history of the injury itself, and the child's course since the injury occurred, should be established from relevant personnel. Any other significant history can be obtained from parents or carers.

Secondary survey

The head should be carefully observed and palpated externally for bruises and lacerations to the scalp and for depressed skull fractures. Look and feel gently inside scalp lacerations for evidence of fractures. Look for evidence of basal skull fracture such as blood or cerebrospinal fluid (CSF) from the nose or ear, haemotympanum, racoon eyes, or Battle's sign (bruising behind the ear, over the mastoid).

The conscious level should be assessed using the relevant Children's Coma Scale if the child is less than 4 years old, and the Glasgow Coma Scale if the child is older than that. These scales are shown in Table 17.1. It should be noted that the Coma Scales reflect the degree of brain dysfunction *at the time of the examination*. Assessment should be repeated frequently.

The pupils should be examined for size and reactivity. A dilated non-reactive pupil indicates third nerve dysfunction; the cause is an ipsilateral haematoma until proven otherwise.

The fundi should be examined using an ophthalmoscope. Papilloedema may not be seen in acute raised intracranial pressure, but the presence of retinal haemorrhage may indicate abuse in a young infant with other unexplained injuries.

Motor function should be assessed. This includes examination of extraocular muscle function, facial and limb movements. Tone, movement, and reflexes should be assessed. Lateralising signs that indicate an intracranial bleed will be revealed in this way.

Investigations

Blood tests

Blood for haemoglobin, urea and electrolytes, and cross-match should have been taken during the primary survey and resuscitation. Arterial blood gases should be taken in head-injured patients, both to assess oxygenation and to measure $Pa\text{co}_2$.

Table 17.1. Glasgow Coma Scale and Children's Coma Scale

Glasgow Coma Scale (4–15 years)		Children's Coma Scale (<4 years)	
Response	Score	Response	Score
Eyes		Eyes	
Open spontaneously	4	Open spontaneously	4
Verbal command	3	React to speech	3
Pain	2	React to pain	2
No response	1	No response	1
Best motor response		Best motor response	
Verbal command:		Spontaneous or obeys verbal	
obeys	6	command	6
Painful stimulus:		*Painful stimulus:*	
Localises pain	5	Localises pain	5
Flexion with pain	4	Withdraws in response to pain	4
		Abnormal flexion to pain	
Flexion abnormal	3	(decorticate posture)	3
		Abnormal extension to pain	
Extension	2	(decerebrate posture)	2
No response	1	No response	1
Best verbal response		Best verbal response	
Orientated and		Smiles, orientated to sounds,	
converse	5	follows objects, interacts	5
Disorientated and		*Crying* *Interacts*	
converse	4	Consolable Inappropriate	4
		Inconsistently	
Inappropriate words	3	consolable Moaning	3
Incomprehensible			
sounds	2	Inconsolable Irritable	2
No response	1	No response No response	1

Radiology

A lateral view of the cervical spine, a chest radiograph, and a radiograph of the pelvis should have been taken during the primary survey.

Skull radiograph In severe head injury a skull radiograph may be superfluous as the information needed will be derived from the CT scan. The role of the skull radiograph in children's head injury is less clear than in adults. In adults the presence of a skull fracture increases the risk of developing a subdural haematoma in the conscious patient from 1:3000 to 1:40. However, in children the test is less specific. Indications for skull radiography are summarised in the box.

Indications for skull radiograph

- Loss of consciousness or amnesia at any time
- Neurological symptoms and signs
- CSF or blood from nose/ear
- Suspected penetrating injury or foreign body
- Scalp bruising or swelling
- Significant mechanism of injury
- Children under 2 years of age with expansile skull sutures
- Difficulty in assessing the patient
- Non-mobile infants (the likelihood of abuse is higher)
- Children in whom an adequate history is not available
- Alcoholic intoxication

154

Computed tomography   CT scanning and neurosurgical referral usually go hand in hand. The exception is the child with a head injury and a Glasgow Coma Score of 14 or less, who is about to undergo life-saving surgery for other serious injuries. A CT scan is indicated in these cases, prior to anaesthetic. Table 17.2 summarises the factors leading to the decision about whether or not to scan.

Table 17.2.   Guidelines for CT scanning of head-injured children

Coma Score	Fracture	Child's condition	CT scan
15	No	No signs	No
15	Yes	No signs	No
15	Yes	Signs/symptoms	Yes
13–14	No	No signs	Consider
13–14	Yes	No signs	Yes
<12	Yes/No	Signs/symptoms +/−	Yes

MANAGEMENT

The initial aim of management of a child with a serious head injury is prevention of secondary brain damage. This is achieved by maintaining ventilation and circulation, and by avoiding raised intracranial pressure.

This can best be achieved by attention to the ABCs discussed earlier. The airway should be secured. Children with a Coma Score of 8 or less should be intubated and ventilated after rapid induction of anaesthesia. This is in order both to maintain full oxygenation and to hyperventilate to a $Pa\text{co}_2$ of approximately 3·7 kPa (28 mmHg). Shock should be treated vigorously to avoid hypoperfusion of the brain.

Analgesia

The withholding of analgesia may contribute to deterioration of the child's condition by leading to a rise in intracranial pressure, and may lead to misinterpretation of the conscious level. Following initial assessment, sufficient analgesia should be administered. Local anaesthetic techniques such as femoral nerve block may be preferable.

Management of specific problems

Deteriorating conscious level
If airway, breathing, and circulation are satisfactory, then a deteriorating conscious level is due to increased intracranial pressure; this may be due either to an intracranial haematoma or to cerebral oedema. Urgent neurosurgical referral is indicated and the temporising manoeuvres shown in the box may be instituted.

Measures to decrease intracranial pressure temporarily

- Nurse in the 30° head-up position
- Hyperventilation to $P\text{co}_2$ of 3·72 kPa (28 mmHg)
- Infusion of intravenous mannitol 0·5–1 g/kg

Signs of uncal or central herniation

These signs (discussed in Chapter 12) should lead to urgent institution of the measures in the box and neurosurgical referral.

Convulsions

A focal seizure should be regarded as a focal neurological sign. A general convulsion has less significance. Seizure activity raises intracranial pressure in both non-paralysed and paralysed patients. The diagnosis is difficult in the latter, but should be suspected if there is a sharp increase in heart rate and blood pressure, and dilatation of the pupils.

Seizures should be controlled if they have not stopped spontaneously within 5 minutes. Phenytoin (18 mg/kg intravenously over 20–30 minutes) should be given, with appropriate monitoring for rhythm irregularities and hypotension.

DEFINITIVE CARE

Neurosurgical referral

Indications for neurosurgical consultation are shown in the box.

Indications for referral to a neurosurgeon

- Deteriorating conscious level
- Focal neurological signs
- Evidence of depressed fracture
- Evidence of penetrating injury
- Evidence of basal skull fracture
- Coma Score of less than 12

Secondary transfer

Transport of critically ill children is usually the responsibility of the referring hospital. It is essential to secure the airway, ensure adequate ventilation, and maintain intravascular volume, temperature, and cerebral perfusion pressure if the child is to arrive in optimum condition. Quality of transfer is better than speed and as much time as necessary should be spent preparing the child (see checklist).

Checklist for transfer

- Adequate sedation
- Full neuromuscular paralysis
- Intermittent positive pressure ventilation (IPPV) preferably by automatic paediatric ventilator
- Oximetry and capnography to monitor ventilation
- Adequate, secure vascular access
- Equipment box
- Heat conservation
- Full medical and nursing notes, charts, and radiographs
- Full parental information

SUMMARY

- Head injury causes primary brain damage. Secondary damage occurs because of the effects of hypoxia, and poor cerebral perfusion
- The first priority is assessment and management of the airway, breathing, and circulation
- A thorough examination including a mini-neurological examination should be carried out during the secondary survey; this involves assessment of external injury, conscious level, pupillary responses, fundi, and motor functions
- Skull radiographs and CT brain scans should be performed if indicated
- The aim of management in the first hour is to prevent secondary damage; this is achieved by attention to airway, breathing, and circulation, and by prompt neurosurgical referral and transfer if indicated

18

Injuries to the extremities and the spine

EXTREMITY TRAUMA

INTRODUCTION

Skeletal injury accounts for 10–15% of all childhood injuries – of these 15% involve physeal disruptions. It is uncommon for extremity trauma to be life threatening in the multiply injured child. It is crucial to recognise and treat associated life-threatening injuries before assessing and managing the skeletal trauma. This chapter deals with problems from the perspective of multiple injury; the principles apply equally to individual injuries.

The differences between the mature and immature skeleton have a bearing on initial treatment and eventual outcome. Use of the principles usually applied to injuries of the mature skeleton will result in errors of both diagnosis and treatment. Unlike the adult skeleton, which is relatively static, the developing skeleton exhibits structural and functional changes, both physiological and biomechanical, which vary throughout growth. These result in different patterns of failure, healing response, and complications.

The two main differences are growth from the physis and the structure of bone. Physeal injury or injury to an epiphyseal ossification centre may result in complete or partial arrest of growth; the latter results in progressive deformity. The relative proportions of lamellar and trabecular bone are constantly changing throughout life and thus result in a change in fracture pattern as the child grows. Up to a certain point children's bones can spring back into shape. As deformation increases, greenstick fractures and then complete fracture occur. The chances of fracture propagation are reduced and comminuted fractures are rare. It should be remembered that children's bones can absorb more force than adults and this may result in an underestimation of the degree of trauma to associated soft tissues.

In the growing child, fracture healing is more rapid and remodelling can occur. Although accurate anatomical alignment should be attempted wherever possible, small degrees of malalignment are acceptable.

ASSESSMENT

Unless extremity injury is life threatening, evaluation is carried out during the secondary survey and treatment commenced during the definitive care phase. Single, closed, extremity injuries may produce enough blood loss to cause hypovolaemic shock, but this is not usually life threatening. Multiple fractures can, however, cause severe shock. Pelvic fractures are relatively uncommon in children – the energy that would have fractured a pelvis in an adult may have been transmitted to vessels within the pelvis of a child, leading to disruption and haemorrhage. Closed fractures of the femur may cause loss of approximately 20% of the intravascular volume into the thigh, and blood loss from open fractures can be even more significant. This blood loss begins at the time of the injury, and it can be difficult to estimate the degree of pre-hospital loss.

Primary survey

All multiply injured children should be approached in the structured way discussed in Chapter 14. Relevant history should be sought from relatives and pre-hospital staff. Extremity deformity and perfusion prior to arrival at hospital are especially important, and information concerning the method of injury is helpful.

Life-threatening injuries
These include the following:

- Crush injuries of the abdomen and pelvis.
- Traumatic amputation of an extremity.
- Massive open long-bone fractures.

They should be dealt with immediately and take precedence over any other extremity injury.

Crush injuries to the abdomen and pelvis Pelvic disruption can lead to life-threatening blood loss. The child will present with hypovolaemic shock; this may remain resistant to treatment until either the pelvic disruption is stabilised or the injured vessels are occluded.

Initial treatment during the primary survey and resuscitation phase consists of rapid fluid and blood infusions as discussed in Chapter 14. The diagnosis may be obvious if disruption is severe or if fractures are open. More often this cause of resistant hypovolaemia is discovered when the pelvic radiograph is taken.

Emergency orthopaedic opinion should be sought, and urgent external fixation of the pelvis should be considered. In some hospitals, radiographic identification and therapeutic embolisation of bleeding vessels may be attempted.

Traumatic amputation Traumatic amputation of an extremity may be partial or complete. Paradoxically, it is usually the former that presents the greatest initial threat to life. This is because completely transected vessels go into spasm whereas partially transected vessels do not. Blood loss can be large and the pre-hospital care of these injuries is critical; an exact history of this should be sought.

Once in hospital the airway should be cleared and breathing assessed as previously discussed. Two wide-bore cannulae should be inserted and rapid crystalloid infusions should be commenced. Exsanguinating haemorrhage must be controlled. If local pressure and elevation are not sufficient, the application of a tourniquet should be considered. If this becomes necessary the tourniquet should be applied as distally as possible, and care should be taken to use a broad rather than a thin cuff. Orthopaedic pneumatic tourniquets are ideal but, if these are not available, a sphygmomanometer cuff inflated to above arterial pressure may be used. The time of application should be recorded, and emergency orthopaedic and plastic surgical opinions sought.

Reimplantation techniques are available in specialist centres. The success rate is improving, particularly in children. Urgent referral and transfer are necessary – the amputated part will only remain viable for 8 hours at room temperature, or for 18 hours if cooled. The amputated part should be cleaned, wrapped in a moist sterile towel, placed in a sterile, sealed plastic bag, and transported in an insulated box filled with crushed ice and water *in the same vehicle as the child*. Care should be taken to avoid direct contact between the ice and tissue.

If, after discussion with the specialist centre, it is decided that reimplantation is not appropriate, the amputated part should still be saved because it may be used for grafting of other injuries.

The child must be stabilised before transfer.

Massive, open, long-bone fractures   The blood loss from any long-bone fractures is significant; open fractures bleed more than closed ones because there is no tamponade effect from surrounding tissues. As a general rule an open fracture causes twice the blood loss of the corresponding closed fracture. Thus a single, open, femoral shaft fracture may result in 40% loss of circulating blood volume. This in itself is life threatening.

After airway and circulation have been assessed and treated, two relatively large-bore cannulae should be inserted and rapid crystalloid infusion should be started. Exsanguinating haemorrhage should be controlled both by the application of pressure at the fracture site, and by correct splinting of the limb.

If haemorrhage cannot be controlled by these techniques, then emergency orthopaedic opinion should be sought. Angiography may be necessary to discover whether any major vessel rupture has occurred, and if such an injury is considered likely then a vascular surgical opinion should be obtained early.

Secondary survey

In a conscious child, inspection is usually the most productive part of the examination. Causing pain or eliciting crepitus in an injured extremity will only increase anxiety, ultimately making the child more difficult to manage.

The extremities should be inspected for discoloration, bruising, swelling, deformity, lacerations, and evidence of open fractures.

Next, *gentle* palpation should be undertaken to establish any areas of tenderness. Limb temperature and capillary refill should be assessed, and pulses sought – a Doppler flow probe should be used if necessary.

Finally, the active range of motion should be assessed if the child is cooperative. If there is an obvious fracture or dislocation, or the child refuses to move a limb actively, passive movement should be avoided.

Limb-threatening injury
The viability of a limb may be threatened by vascular injury, compartment syndrome, or by open fractures. These situations are discussed below.

Vascular injury   Assessment of the vascular status of the extremity is a vital step in evaluating an injury. Vascular damage may be caused by traction (resulting in intimal damage or complete disruption), or by penetrating injuries caused by either a missile or the end of a fractured bone. Brisk bleeding from an open wound or a rapidly expanding mass is indicative of active bleeding. Complete tears are less likely to bleed for a prolonged period due to contraction of the vessel. It should be remembered that nerves usually pass in close proximity to vessels and are likely to have been damaged along with the vessel.

The presence of a pulse, either clinically or on Doppler examination, does not rule out a vascular injury. *A diminished pulse should not be attributed to spasm.*

The signs of vascular injury are shown in the box.

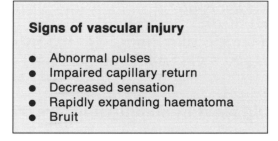

Signs of vascular injury

- Abnormal pulses
- Impaired capillary return
- Decreased sensation
- Rapidly expanding haematoma
- Bruit

If these signs are present, urgent investigation and management should be commenced. The fracture should be aligned and splints checked to ensure that they are not restrictive; if no improvement occurs a vascular surgeon should be consulted and angiography considered. Vascular damage may not always be immediately apparent; constant reassessment is therefore essential.

Compartment syndrome If the interstitial pressure within a fascial compartment rises above capillary pressure, then local muscle ischaemia occurs. If this is unrecognised, it eventually results in Volkmann's ischaemic contracture.

Compartment syndrome usually develops over a period of hours and is most often associated with crush injuries. It may, however, occur following simple fractures. The classic signs are shown in the box.

Classic signs of compartment syndrome

- Pain, accentuated by passively stretching the involved muscles
- Decreased sensation
- Swelling
- Weakness

Distal pulses only disappear when the intracompartmental pressure rises above arterial pressure; by this time irreversible changes have usually occurred in the muscle bed. Initial treatment consists of releasing constricting bandages and splints. If this is ineffective then urgent surgical fasciotomy should be performed.

Open fractures

**Any wound within the vicinity of a fracture should
be assumed to communicate with the fracture.**

Open wounds are classified according to the degree of soft tissue damage, amount of contamination, and the presence or absence of associated neurovascular damage. Initial treatment includes removal of gross contamination, and covering of the wound with a sterile dressing. No attempt should be made to ligate bleeding points because associated nerves may be damaged as this is done. Bleeding should be controlled by direct pressure.

Broad-spectrum antibiotics should be given, and tetanus immunisation status checked. Further management is surgical – débridement should be carried out within 8 hours.

Other injuries

Non-accidental injury
This must always be considered if the history is not consistent with the injury pattern. It is discussed in detail in Appendix C.

Fracture–dislocation
It is difficult to distinguish fractures and fracture–dislocations on clinical grounds. Radiology is often helpful, but in very young children, where ossification centres have not yet formed, an ultrasound examination or arthrogram may be necessary. In an older child (when some of the ossification centres are present), a comparative radiograph of the normal side may be helpful before more invasive investigations are considered. These investigations should be performed in the definitive care phase, unless there are vascular or neurological complications.

Dislocations
Dislocations, other than of the elbow and hip, are rare in children but, as for adults, may produce neurovascular injury that can result in permanent impairment. All dislocations should therefore be reduced as soon as possible.

Epiphyseal injuries
Fractures involving the epiphysis may be displaced or non-displaced. They should be managed by an orthopaedic surgeon.

MANAGEMENT

Life-threatening problems identified during the primary survey in the multiply injured patient are managed first. Only then should attention be turned to the extremity injury. The specific management of complications such as vascular injury, compartment syndrome, traumatic amputation, and open wounds have been discussed earlier in this chapter.

Alignment

Severely angulated fractures should be aligned. Gentle traction should be applied to the limb to facilitate alignment, particularly when immobilising long-bone fractures. Splints should extend one joint above and below the fracture site. Perfusion of the extremity, including pulses, skin colour, temperature, and neurological status, must be assessed before and after the fracture is aligned. Radiographs, including arteriograms, should *not* be obtained until the extremity is splinted.

When aligning a fracture, analgesia is usually necessary. Entonox or intravenous opiates should be used. In femoral fractures, femoral nerve block is very effective – the technique is discussed in Chapter 23.

Immobilisation

Fractures (or suspected fractures) should be immobilised to control pain and prevent further injury. Splintage is a most effective way of controlling pain and subsequent doses of analgesia may be reduced. If pain increases after immobilisation, then an ischaemic injury and/or compartment syndrome must be excluded. Emergency splinting techniques for various injured extremities are described below.

163

Upper limb
Hand   Splinted in the position of function with the wrist slightly dorsiflexed and the fingers slightly flexed at all joints. This is best achieved by gently immobilising the hand over a large roll of gauze.

Forearm and wrist   Splinted flat on padded pillows or splints.

Elbow   Immobilised in a flexed position with a sling which may be strapped to the body.

Arm   Immobilised by a sling, which can be augmented with splints for unstable fractures. Circumferential bandages should be avoided as they may be the cause of constriction, particularly when swelling occurs.

Shoulder   Immobilised by a sling.

Lower limb
Femur   Femoral fractures should be treated in traction splints. Ipsilateral femoral and tibial fractures can be immobilised in the same splint. Excess traction may cause perineal injury and neurovascular problems, and should be avoided.

Tibia and ankle   Tibial and ankle fractures should be aligned and immobilised in padded box splints. Foot perfusion should be assessed before and after application of the splint.

SUMMARY

- Extremity trauma is rarely life threatening per se, unless exsanguinating haemorrhage ensues. Multiple fractures can cause significant blood loss
- The first priority is assessment of the airway, breathing, and circulation
- Full assessment of the extremities takes place during the secondary survey. Limb-threatening injuries should be identified at this stage and further investigation and management begun. Other injuries should be treated by splintage

SPINAL TRAUMA

Spinal injuries are rare in children which does not mean that they are unimportant. A high index of suspicion, correct management, and prompt referral are necessary in order to prevent exacerbation of underlying cord injury. Every severely injured child should be treated as though he or she has spinal injury until adequate examination and investigation exclude it.

INJURIES OF THE CERVICAL SPINE

Injuries to the cervical spine are rare in children. The upper three vertebrae are usually involved – injury is more common in the lower segments of an adult. The low incidence (0·2% of all children's fractures and dislocations) of bony injury is explained by the

164

mobility of the cervical spine in children, which dissipates applied forces over a greater number of segments.

Radiographs

A lateral cervical spine radiograph will have been obtained during the primary survey. Injury must be presumed until excluded radiologically and clinically. Spinal injury may be present even with a normal radiograph. The development of the cervical vertebrae is complex. There are numerous physeal lines (which can be confused with fractures), and a range of normal sites for ossification centres. Pseudosubluxation of C2 on C3 and of C3 on C4 occurs in approximately 9% of children, particularly those aged 1–7 years. Interpretation of cervical radiographs can therefore be difficult even for the most experienced.

Indirect evidence of trauma can be detected by assessing retropharyngeal swelling. At the inferior part of the body of C3, the prevertebral distance should be two-thirds the width of the body of C2. This distance varies during breathing and is increased in a crying child.

Injury types

Atlantoaxial rotary subluxation is the most common injury to the cervical spine. The child presents with torticollis following trauma. Radiological demonstration of the injury is difficult, and computed tomography or magnetic resonance imaging may be necessary. Other injuries of C1 and C2 include odontoid epiphyseal separations and traumatic ligament disruption. Injuries below C2 are particularly rare.

It should be noted that significant cervical cord injuries have been reported without any radiological evidence of trauma.

Immediate treatment

Despite the rarity of fractures a severely injured child's spine should be securely immobilised until orthopaedic or neurosurgical advice has been obtained.

Cervical spine immobilisation techniques are described in Chapter 23.

INJURIES OF THE THORACIC AND LUMBAR SPINE

Injuries to the thoracic and lumbar spine are rare in children and account for less than 1% of all spinal injuries. They are most common in the multiply injured child. In the second decade, 44% of reported injuries result from sporting and other recreational activity. Some spinal injuries may result from non-accidental injury.

When an injury does occur, it is not uncommon to find multiple levels of involvement because the force is dissipated over many segments in the child's mobile spine. This increased mobility may also lead to neurological involvement without significant skeletal injury.

The most common mechanism of injury is hyperflexion and the most common radiographic finding is a wedge- or beak-shaped vertebra resulting from compression.

The most important clinical sign is a sensory level. Neurological assessment is difficult in children, and such a level may only become apparent after repeated examinations. Because of the difficulties of assessment, a child with multiple injuries should be assumed to have spinal injury, and should therefore be immobilised on a long spine board until investigations and examinations are complete. If injury is confirmed, further treatment is similar to that in adults. Unstable injuries may require open reduction and stabilisation with fusion.

If cord damage does occur, children can suffer the same complications as adults. In addition, late, progressive deformity to the spine may occur secondary to differential growth occurring around the injured segments.

SUMMARY

- Spinal injuries are rare in children
- Assessment can be difficult and significant cord damage can occur without fractures
- Spinal immobilisation must be applied until such time as assessment is complete

19

Burns

INTRODUCTION

Epidemiology

Each year some 20 000 burnt and 30 000 scalded children attend accident and emergency departments. Of these, 5000–6000 require hospital admission. In England and Wales in 1989, 90 children died from burns, and 5 from scalds. Seventy per cent of those burnt are pre-school children, the most common age being between 1 and 2 years. Scalds occur mostly in the under-4s. Boys are more likely to suffer burns and serious scalds.

Most fatal burns occur in house fires and smoke inhalation is the usual cause of death. The number of deaths from burns have decreased because of a combination of factors. The move away from open fires, safer fireguards, and more stringent low flammability requirements for night clothes have all played a part. Non-fatal burns often involve clothing and are often associated with flammable liquids. They show no sign of decreasing in number.

Scalds are usually caused by hot drinks, but bath water and cooking oil scalds are not uncommon. The improvement in survival following scalding (which followed improvements in treatment) has reached a plateau.

There is a strong link between burns to children and low socioeconomic status. Family stress, poor housing conditions, and over-crowding are implicated in this.

Pathophysiology

Two main factors determine the severity of burns and scalds – these are the temperature and the duration of contact. The time taken for cellular destruction to occur decreases exponentially with temperature. At 44°C, contact would have to be maintained for 6 hours, at 54°C for 30 seconds, and at 70°C epidermal injury happens within a second. This relationship underlies the different patterns of injury seen with different types of burn. Scalds generally involve water at below boiling point and contact for less than 4 seconds. Scalds that occur with liquids at a higher temperature (such as hot fat), or in children incapable of minimising the contact time (such as young infants and the handicapped), tend to result in more serious injuries. Flame burns can involve high temperatures and prolonged contact and consequently produce the most serious injuries of all.

It must be re-emphasised that the most common cause of death within the first hour following burn injuries is smoke inhalation. Thus, as with other types of injury, attention to the airway and breathing is of prime importance.

PRIMARY SURVEY AND RESUSCITATION

When faced with a seriously burnt child it is easy to focus on the immediate problems of the burn, and forget the possibility of other injuries. The approach to the burnt child should be the structured one advocated in Chapter 14.

Airway and cervical spine

The airway may be compromised either because of inhalational injury, or because of severe burns to the face. The latter are usually obvious whereas the former may only be indicated more subtly. The indicators of inhalational injury are shown in the box.

Indications of inhalational injury

- History of exposure to smoke in a confined space
- Deposits around the mouth and nose
- Carbonaceous sputum

Since oedema occurs following thermal injury, the airway can deteriorate rapidly. Thus even suspicion of airway compromise, or the discovery of injuries that might be expected to cause problems with the airway at a later stage, should lead to immediate consideration of endotracheal intubation. This procedure increases in difficulty as oedema progresses, and it is important to perform it as soon as possible. All but the most experienced should seek expert help urgently, unless apnoea requires immediate intervention.

If there is any suspicion of cervical spine injury, or if the history is unobtainable, appropriate precautions should be taken until such injury is excluded.

Breathing

Once the airway has been secured, the adequacy of breathing should be assessed. Signs that should arouse suspicion of inadequacy include: abnormal rate, abnormal chest movements, and cyanosis (a late sign). Circumferential burns to the chest may cause breathing difficulty by mechanically restricting chest movement.

All children who have suffered burns should be given high-flow oxygen. If there are signs of breathing problems then ventilation should be commenced.

Circulation

In the first few hours following injury signs of hypovolaemic shock are rarely attributable to burns. Therefore any such signs should raise the suspicion of bleeding from elsewhere, and the source should be actively sought. Intravenous access should be established with two cannulae during resuscitation and fluids started. If possible drips should be put up in unburnt areas, but eschar can be perforated if necessary. Remember that the intraosseous route can be used. Blood should be taken for haemoglobin, haematocrit, electrolytes and urea, and cross-matching at this stage.

Disability

Reduced conscious level following burns may be due to hypoxia (following smoke inhalation), head injury, or hypovolaemia. It is essential that a quick assessment is made during the primary survey as described in Chapter 14, because this provides a baseline for later observations.

Exposure

Exposure should be complete. Burnt children lose heat especially rapidly, and must be covered with blankets when not being examined.

SECONDARY SURVEY

As well as being burnt, children may suffer the effects of blast, may be injured by falling objects, and may fall while trying to escape from the fire. Thus other injuries are not uncommon and a thorough head-to-toe secondary survey should be carried out. This is described in Chapter 14. Any injuries discovered, including the burn, should be treated in order of priority.

Assessing the burn

The severity of a burn depends on its relative surface area and depth. Burns to particular areas may require special care.

Surface area

The surface area is usually estimated using burns charts. It is particularly important to use a paediatric chart when assessing burn size in children, because the relative surface areas of the head and limbs change with age. This variation is illustrated in Figure 19.1 and its accompanying table.

Another useful method of estimating relative surface area relies on the fact that the patient's palm and adducted fingers cover an area of approximately 1% of the body surface. This method can be used when charts are not immediately available, and is obviously already related to the child's size.

Note that the "rule of nines" cannot be applied to a child who is less than 14 years old.

Depth

Burns are classified as being superficial, partial thickness, or full thickness. The first causes injury only to the epidermis and clinically the skin appears red with no blister formation. Partial-thickness burns cause some damage to the dermis; blistering is usually seen and the skin is pink or mottled. Deeper (full-thickness) burns damage both the epidermis and dermis, and may cause injury to deeper structures as well. The skin looks white or charred, and is painless and leathery to touch.

Special areas

Burns to the face and mouth have already been dealt with above. Burns involving the hand can cause severe functional loss if scarring occurs. Perineal burns are prone to infection and present particularly difficult management problems.

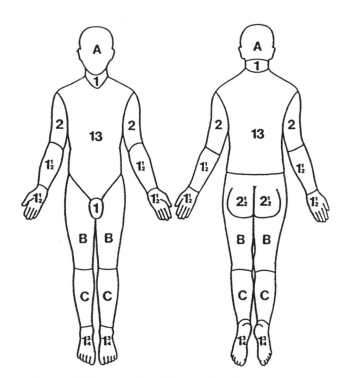

Figure 19.1. Lund and Browder charts

Area indicated	Surface area at				
	0	1 year	5 years	10 years	15 years
A	9·5	8·5	6·5	5·5	4·5
B	2·75	3·25	4·0	4·5	4·5
C	2·5	2·5	2·75	3·0	3·25

INITIAL BURN CARE

Analgesia

Most burnt children will be in severe pain, and this should be dealt with urgently. Some older children may manage to use Entonox, but most will not. Any child with burns that are anything other than minor should be given *intravenous* morphine at a dose of 0·1 mg/kg as soon as possible. There is no place for administration of intramuscular analgesia in severe burns because absorption is unreliable.

Fluid therapy

Two cannulae should already have been sited during the primary survey and resuscitation, and therapy for shock (20 ml/kg) commenced if indicated. Children with burns of 10% or more will require intravenous fluids as part of their burns care, in addition to their normal fluid requirement. The *additional* fluid (in ml) required per day to treat the burn can be estimated using the following formula:

$$\text{Percentage burn} \times \text{Weight (kg)} \times 4$$

and of this half should be given in the first 8 hours *since the time of their burn*. The fluid given is usually 4·5% human albumin. Remember that this is only an initial guide. Subsequent therapy will be guided by urine output, which should be kept at 1 ml/kg/h or more. Urethral catheterisation should therefore be performed as soon as is practicable.

Wound care

Infection is a significant cause of mortality and morbidity in burns victims, and wound care should start as early as possible to reduce this risk. Furthermore, appropriate wound care will reduce the pain associated with air passing over burnt areas.

Burns should be covered with sterile towels, and unnecessary re-examination should be avoided. Blisters should be left intact. Although cold compresses and irrigation with cold water may reduce pain, it should be remembered that burnt children lose heat rapidly. These treatments should only be used for 10 minutes or less, and only in patients with partial-thickness burns totalling less than 10%. Children should *never* be transferred with cold soaks in place.

DEFINITIVE CARE

Definitive care requires transfer to a paediatric burns facility. Criteria for transfer are shown in the box.

Criteria for transfer to a burns unit

- 10% partial- and/or full-thickness burns
- 5% full-thickness burns
- Burns to special areas

If in doubt discuss the child with the paediatric burns unit.

SUMMARY

- Initial assessment and management of the burnt child should be directed towards care of the airway, breathing, and circulation. Intubation and ventilation should be performed early if indicated
- Assessment of the area and depth of the burn should be undertaken during the secondary survey
- Fluid replacement should be used initially to treat shock. Additional fluids will be needed to treat the burn, and a guide to the amount required can be calculated. Urine output should be used as an indicator of the efficacy of treatment
- Specialist burns centres should be contacted, and transfer arranged if indicated

---

20

Electrical injuries and near drowning

ELECTRICAL INJURIES

INTRODUCTION

Epidemiology

Children account for 33% of all victims of electrical injuries; approximately 20% of reported electrical injuries are fatal. Over 90% result from accidents involving generated electricity.

Pathophysiology

The following factors determine the effects of an electric shock.

Current

Alternating current (AC) produces cardiac arrest at lower voltage than does direct current (DC). Whether electrocution is with AC or DC, the risk of cardiac arrest is greater with increasing size and duration of current passing through the heart; the current will be greater with low resistance and high voltage.

Lightning acts as a massive DC countershock which depolarises the myocardium and may lead to immediate asystole and death.

As current increases the effects listed in the box may be seen.

Effect of increase in current

Above 10 mA: tetanic contractions of muscles may make it impossible for the child to let go of the electrical source

50 mA: tetanic contraction of the diaphragm and intercostal muscles leads to respiratory arrest which continues until the current is disconnected. If hypoxia is prolonged, secondary cardiac arrest will occur

Over 100 mA to several amps: primary cardiac arrest may be induced (defibrillators used in resuscitation deliver around 10 A)

50 A to hundreds of amps: massive shocks cause prolonged respiratory and cardiac arrest, and more severe burns

---

Resistance

The resistance of tissues determines the path that the current follows. In general this is the path of least resistance from the entry point on the victim to the ground. Thus current preferentially flows down nerves and blood vessels, rather than through muscles, skin, tendon, fat, or bone. Electrocution of tissues with high resistance will generate most heat, and tissues tolerate this to varying degrees. Overall, nerves, blood vessels, skin, and muscle sustain most injury.

Water reduces skin resistance and thereby increases the current delivered to the body.

Voltage

High voltage ("tension") sources such as overhead electric power lines or lightning involve a higher current, and consequently cause more tissue damage than lower voltage sources.

MANAGEMENT

Prior to commencing treatment it is essential that the child is disconnected from the electric source.

Primary survey and resuscitation

The airway may be compromised by facial burns, and early management of such problems is essential (see Chapter 19). If the child is unconscious, the neck should be assumed to be broken and must be protected until injury is excluded. Other life-threatening injuries may occur during secondary trauma and must be treated appropriately.

Secondary survey

Virtually any injury can occur. In particular, associated injuries can arise from being thrown from the source. Burns are common, and happen either because of the direct effects of the current (exit burns are often more severe than entry burns), or secondary to the ignition of clothing. The powerful tetanic contraction caused by the shock can cause fractures, dislocations, or muscle tearing.

LATE COMPLICATIONS

Cutaneous and deep tissue burns lead to fluid loss and oedema with dehydration. Myoglobinuria may arise if there is significant muscle breakdown. In such cases acute renal failure is a very real threat and a forced diuresis of *at least* 2 ml/kg/h must be maintained. Metabolic acidosis must be corrected with intravenous sodium bicarbonate because myoglobin is more soluble in alkaline urine.

REFERRAL

All children suffering from electrical burns should be discussed with the local Burns Unit; transfer to such specialist centres is usually indicated.

SUMMARY

- Cardiorespiratory arrest can occur
- Associated injuries may arise as a result of being thrown from the source
- Electrical burns may cause significant damage to deep structures. The extent of this damage may not be apparent on external examination
- All electrical burns should be discussed with burns centres

NEAR DROWNING

INTRODUCTION

Drowning is defined as death from asphyxia associated with submersion in a fluid. Near drowning is said to have occurred if there is any recovery (however transient) following a submersion incident.

Epidemiology

The incidence of near drowning is unknown, but drowning is the third most common cause of accidental death in children in the UK (after road accidents and burns). In England and Wales the annual incidence of submersion accidents in under 15 year olds is 1·5 per 100 000 and the mortality in this age group is 0·7 per 100 000. The highest incidence (3·6 per 100 000) occurs in boys under 5 years old. Children most commonly die in private swimming pools, garden ponds, and other inland waterways.

Pathophysiology

When a child is first submerged, breath-holding occurs and the heart rate slows because of the diving reflex. As apnoea continues hypoxia causes tachycardia, a rise in the blood pressure, and acidosis. Between 20 seconds and 2·5 minutes later a break point is reached, and breathing occurs. Fluid is inhaled and on touching the glottis causes immediate laryngeal spasm. Secondary apnoea eventually gives way to involuntary respiratory movements, and water, weeds, and debris enter the lungs. Bradycardia and arrhythmias follow, heralding cardiac arrest and death.

Children who survive because of interruption of this chain of events not only require therapy for near drowning, but also assessment and treatment of concomitant hypothermia, electrolyte imbalance, and injury (particularly spinal).

MANAGEMENT

Primary survey and resuscitation

The neck must be presumed to be injured, and the cervical spine should be immobilised until such injury is excluded. A history of diving is especially significant in this regard.

Following a significant near-drowning episode, the stomach is usually full of swallowed water. The risk of aspiration is therefore increased and tracheal intubation and gastric decompression must be performed early to protect the airway.

175

A core temperature reading must be obtained as soon as possible. Hypothermia is common following near drowning, and adversely affects resuscitation attempts unless treated. Not only are arrhythmias more common but some, such as ventricular fibrillation, may be refractory at temperatures below 30°C. Resuscitation should not be discontinued until core temperature is at least 32°C.

Rewarming

External rewarming is usually sufficient if core temperature is above 32°C. Active core rewarming should be added in patients with a core temperature of less than 32°C, but beware "rewarming shock", which may result from hypovolaemia becoming apparent during peripheral vasodilatation. External and internal rewarming methods are shown in the box.

External rewarming

- Remove cold, wet clothing
- Apply warm blankets
- Infrared radiant lamp
- Heating blanket

Core rewarming

- Warm intravenous fluids to 37°C
- Warm ventilator gases to 42°C
- Gastric or bladder lavage with normal (physiological) saline at 42°C
- Peritoneal lavage with potassium-free dialysate at 42°C. Use 20 ml/kg cycled every 15 minutes
- Pleural or pericardial lavage
- Extracorporeal blood rewarming

Rhythm, pulse rate, and blood pressure monitoring should be undertaken.

Secondary survey

During the secondary survey, the child should be carefully examined from head to toe. Any injury may have occurred during the incident that preceded submersion; spinal injuries are particularly common.

Investigations

- Blood glucose.
- Arterial blood gases.
- Electrolytes.
- Baseline chest radiograph.
- Blood cultures.

Definitive care

Fever is common in the first few hours, but systemic infection should be suspected if a pyrexia develops after 24 hours. Once blood cultures have been taken, intravenous antibiotics can be started. The chosen agent should be effective against Gram-negative organisms. In children penicillin and cefotaxime are used. Regular tracheal cultures, blood cultures, electrolytes, and white cell counts should be taken.

PROGNOSTIC INDICATORS

Immersion time

Most children who do not recover have been submerged for more than 3–8 minutes. Details of the rescue are therefore vital.

Time to first gasp

If this occurs between 1 and 3 minutes after the start of basic cardiopulmonary support, the prognosis is good. If there has been no gasp after 40 minutes of full cardiopulmonary resuscitation, there is little or no chance of survival unless the child's respiration has been depressed (for example, by hypothermia or alcohol).

Rectal temperature

If this is less than 33°C on arrival, the chances of survival are increased because rapid cooling protects vital organs. Children cool quickly because of their large surface area/volume ratio.

Persisting coma

This indicates a bad prognosis.

Arterial blood pH

If this remains less than 7·0 despite treatment, the prognosis is poor.

Arterial blood PO_2

If this remains less than 8·0 kPa (60 mmHg), despite treatment, the prognosis is poor.

Type of water

Whether the water was salt or fresh has no bearing on the prognosis.

The decision to discontinue resuscitation attempts is particularly difficult in cases of drowning, and should be taken only after all the prognostic factors discussed above have been considered carefully.

OUTCOME

Seventy per cent of children survive near drowning when basic life support is provided at the waterside. Only 40% survive without early basic life support even if full advanced cardiopulmonary resuscitation is given in hospital.

Of those who do survive, having required full cardiopulmonary resuscitation in hospital, around 70% will make a complete recovery and 25% will have a mild neurological deficit. The remainder will be severely disabled or remain in a persisting vegetative state.

SUMMARY

- There is a high incidence of associated cervical spine injury especially during diving accidents
- Other associated injuries may arise during the incident leading to submersion
- Hypothermia should be actively sought and treated
- Resuscitation attempts must not be abandoned until the core temperature is at least 32°C

PRACTICAL PROCEDURES

21

Procedures – airway and breathing

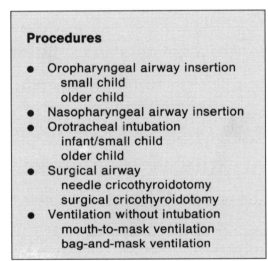

Procedures

- Oropharyngeal airway insertion
  small child
  older child
- Nasopharyngeal airway insertion
- Orotracheal intubation
  infant/small child
  older child
- Surgical airway
  needle cricothyroidotomy
  surgical cricothyroidotomy
- Ventilation without intubation
  mouth-to-mask ventilation
  bag-and-mask ventilation

OROPHARYNGEAL AIRWAY INSERTION

If the gag reflex is present, it may be best to avoid the use of an oropharyngeal tube or other artificial airway, because it may cause choking, laryngospasm, or vomiting.

Small child

1. Select an appropriately sized Guedel airway.
2. Open the airway using the chin lift, taking care not to move the neck if trauma has occurred.
3. Use a tongue depressor or a laryngoscope blade to aid insertion of the airway "the right way up" (Figure 21.1).
4. Re-check airway patency.
5. If necessary, consider a different size from the original estimate.
6. Finally provide oxygen, consider ventilation by pocket mask or bag and mask.

Older child

1. Select an appropriately sized Guedel airway.
2. Open the airway using the chin lift, taking care not to move the neck if trauma has occurred.
3. Insert the airway concave upwards until the tip reaches the soft palate.
4. Rotate it through 180° (concave side downwards) and slide it back over the tongue.
5. Re-check airway patency.
6. If necessary, consider a different size from the original estimate.
7. Finally provide oxygen, consider ventilation by pocket mask or bag and mask.

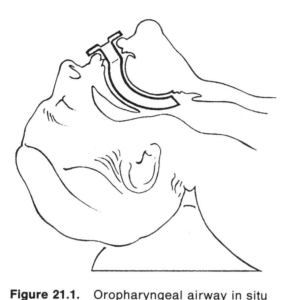

Figure 21.1. Oropharyngeal airway in situ

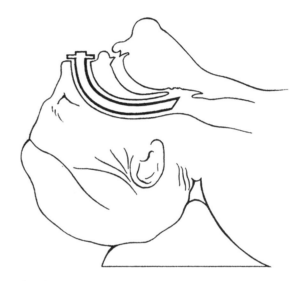

Figure 21.2. Nasopharyngeal airway in situ

NASOPHARYNGEAL AIRWAY INSERTION

Assess for any contraindications such as a base of skull fracture.

1. Select an appropriate size (length and diameter).
2. Lubricate the airway with a water-soluble lubricant, and insert a large safety pin through the flange.
3. Insert the tip into the nostril and direct it posteriorly along the floor of the nose (rather than upwards).
4. Gently pass the airway past the turbinates with a slight rotating motion. As the tip advances into the pharynx, there should be a palpable "give".
5. Continue until the flange and safety pin rest on the nostril (Figure 21.2).
6. If there is difficulty inserting the airway, consider using the other nostril or a smaller size from the original estimate.
7. Re-check airway patency.
8. Finally provide oxygen, consider ventilation by pocket mask or bag and mask.

OROTRACHEAL INTUBATION

Infant or small child

1. Ensure that adequate ventilation and oxygenation by face mask are in progress.
2. Select an appropriate laryngoscope, and check the brightness of the light.

3. Select an appropriate tube size, but prepare a range of sizes, including the size above and below the best estimate.
4. Ensure manual immobilisation of the neck by an assistant if cervical spine injury is possible. Because of the relatively large occiput, it may be helpful to place a folded sheet or towel under the baby's back and neck to allow extension of the head. In the delivery suite, the design of the Resuscitaire allows the neonate's head to rest in the correct position (Figure 21.3).

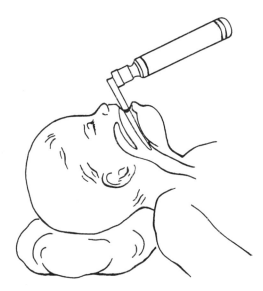

Figure 21.3. Orotracheal intubation – straight-blade laryngoscope technique

5. Hold the laryngoscope in the left hand, and insert it into the right-hand side of the mouth, displacing the tongue to the left. In the infant, it is sometimes useful to hold the laryngoscope with the left thumb, and index and middle fingers, leaving the little finger free to stretch down to press on the larynx to improve the view of the vocal cords (vocal folds). This is particularly useful if single handed.
6. In the "flat" baby being intubated by a relatively inexperienced doctor, it is often easiest to place the laryngoscope blade well beyond the epiglottis. The laryngoscope blade is placed down the right-hand side of the tongue into the proximal oesophagus. With a careful lifting movement, the tissues are gently tented up to "seek the midline". The blade is then slowly withdrawn until the vocal cords come into view. In some situations, it may be better to stay proximal to the epiglottis to minimise the risk of causing laryngospasm. This decision must be based on clinical judgement.
7. Insert the endotracheal tube into the trachea, concentrating on how far the tip is being placed below the vocal cords. The tip should lie 2–4 cm below the vocal cords depending on age. If the tube has a "vocal cord level" marker, place this at the vocal cords. Be aware that flexion or extension of the neck may cause migration downwards or upwards, respectively.
8. Check the placement of the tube by inspecting the chest for movement and auscultating the chest (including the axillae) and epigastrium.
9. If endotracheal intubation is not achieved in 30 seconds, discontinue the attempt, ventilate and oxygenate by mask, and try again.
10. Once the tube is in place obtain a chest radiograph to confirm correct placement.

Older child

1. Ensure that adequate ventilation and oxygenation by face mask are in progress.
2. Select an appropriate laryngoscope, and check the brightness of the light.
3. Select an appropriate tube size, but prepare a range of sizes, including the size above and below the best estimate.
4. Ensure manual immobilisation of the neck by an assistant if cervical spine injury is possible.
5. Hold the laryngoscope in the left hand, and insert it into the right-hand side of the mouth, displacing the tongue to the left.
6. Visualise the epiglottis, and place the tip of the laryngoscope in the vallecula.
7. Gently but firmly lift the handle "towards the ceiling on the far side of the room", being careful not to lever on the teeth (Figure 21.4).

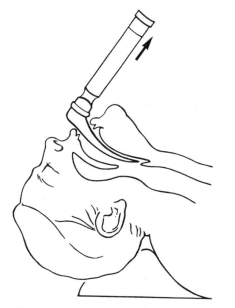

Figure 21.4. Orotracheal intubation – curved-blade laryngoscope technique

8. Insert the endotracheal tube into the trachea, concentrating on how far the tip is being placed below the vocal cords (vocal folds). The tip should lie 2–4 cm below the vocal cords depending on age. If the tube has a "vocal cord level" marker, place this at the vocal cords. Be aware that flexion or extension of the neck may cause migration downwards or upwards, respectively.
9. In the adolescent, inflate the cuff to provide an adequate seal. In the pre-pubertal child do not use a cuffed tube.
10. Check the placement of the tube by inspecting the chest for movement and auscultating the chest (including the axillae) and epigastrium.
11. If endotracheal intubation is not achieved in 30 seconds, discontinue the attempt, ventilate and oxygenate by mask, and try again.
12. Once the tube is in place obtain a chest radiograph to confirm correct placement.

Complications of endotracheal intubation
These include:

-   Oesophageal intubation (causing severe hypoxia if not immediately recognised).
-   Endobronchial intubation, resulting in lung collapse and risk of pneumothorax.
-   Severe hypoxia from a prolonged attempt to intubate.

- Airway injury from the laryngoscope, tube, or stylet (including direct trauma to the vocal cords), as well as chipping or loosening of the teeth.
- Neck strain by overextension, or exacerbation of a cervical spine injury with risk of neurological deterioration.

SURGICAL AIRWAY

Cricothyroidotomy is a "technique of failure". It is indicated if a patent airway cannot be achieved by other means. It must be performed promptly and decisively when necessary.

In children under the age of 12 years, needle cricothyroidotomy is preferred to surgical cricothyroidotomy. In the adolescent either technique can be used but the surgical technique allows better protection of the airway. The relevant anatomy is shown in Figure 21.5.

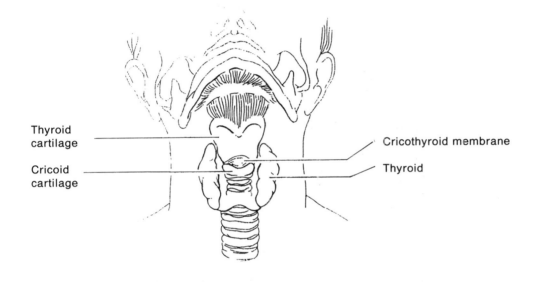

Thyroid cartilage

Cricoid cartilage

Cricothyroid membrane

Thyroid

Figure 21.5. Surgical airway – relevant anatomy

In a very small baby, or if a foreign body is below the cricoid ring, direct tracheal puncture using the same technique can be used.

Needle cricothyroidotomy

This technique is simple in concept, but far from easy in practice. In an emergency situation the child may be struggling, and attempts to breathe or swallow may result in the larynx moving up and down:

1. Attach a cricothyroidotomy cannula-over-needle (or if not available, an intravenous cannula and needle) of appropriate size to a 5 ml syringe.
2. Place the patient in a supine position.
3. If there is no risk of cervical spine injury, extend the neck, perhaps with a sandbag under the shoulders.
4. Identify the cricothyroid membrane by palpation between the thyroid and cricoid cartilages.
5. Prepare the neck with antiseptic swabs.

185

6. Place your left hand on the neck to identify and stabilise the cricothyroid membrane, and to protect the lateral vascular structures from needle injury.
7. Insert the needle and cannula through the cricothyroid membrane at a 45° angle caudally, aspirating as the needle is advanced (Figure 21.6).

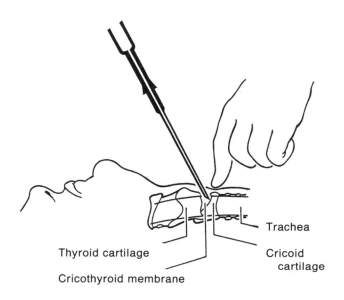

Trachea

Thyroid cartilage

Cricoid cartilage

Cricothyroid membrane

Figure 21.6. Needle cricothyroidotomy

8. When air is aspirated, advance the cannula over the needle, being careful not to damage the posterior tracheal wall. Withdraw the needle.
9. Re-check that air can be aspirated from the cannula.
10. Attach the hub of the cannula to an oxygen flowmeter via a Y-connector. Initially the oxygen flow rate (in litres) should be set at the child's age (in years).
11. Ventilate by occluding the open end of the Y-connector with a thumb for 1 second, to direct gas into the lungs. If this does not cause the chest to rise the oxygen flow rate should be increased by increments of 1 litre, and the effect of 1 second's occlusion of the Y-connector reassessed.

Important notes

There are two common misconceptions about transtracheal insufflation. The first is that it is possible to ventilate a patient via a needle cricothyroidotomy using a self-inflating bag. The maximum pressure from a bag is approximately 4·41 kPa (45 cmH$_2$O) (the blow-off valve pressure) and this is insufficient to drive gas through a narrow cannula. In comparison, wall oxygen is provided at a pressure of 4 atmospheres (approximately 392 kPa or 4000 cmH$_2$O). The second misconception is that expiration can occur through the cannula, or through a separate cannula inserted through the cricothyroid membrane. This is not possible. The intratracheal pressure during expiration is usually less than 2·9 kPa (30 cmH$_2$O) (less than one-hundredth of the driving pressure in inspiration). Expiration must occur via the upper airway, even in situations of partial upper airway obstruction. Should upper airway obstruction be complete, it is necessary to reduce the gas flow to 1–2 l/min. This provides some oxygenation but little ventilation.
  Nevertheless, insufflation buys a few minutes in which to attempt a surgical airway.

12. Allow passive exhalation (via the upper airway) by taking the thumb off for 4 seconds.
13. Observe chest movement and auscultate breath sounds to confirm adequate ventilation.
14. Check the neck to exclude swelling from the injection of gas into the tissues rather than the trachea.
15. Secure the equipment to the patient's neck.
16. Having completed emergency airway management, arrange to proceed to a more definitive airway procedure, such as tracheotomy.

Surgical cricothyroidotomy

This should only be considered in the older child (12 years or over):

1. Place the patient in a supine position.
2. If there is no risk of neck injury, consider extending the neck to improve access. Otherwise, maintain a neutral alignment.
3. Identify the cricothyroid membrane.
4. Prepare the skin and, if the patient is conscious, infiltrate with local anaesthetic.
5. Place your left hand on the neck to stabilise the cricothyroid membrane, and to protect the lateral vascular structures from injury.
6. Make a small vertical incision in the skin, and press the lateral edges of the incision outwards, to minimise bleeding.
7. Make a transverse incision through the cricothyroid membrane, being careful not to damage the cricoid cartilage.
8. Insert a tracheal spreader, or use the handle of the scalpel by inserting it through the incision and twisting it through 90° to open the airway.
9. Insert an appropriately sized endotracheal or tracheostomy tube. It is advisable to use a slightly smaller size than would have been used for an oral or nasal tube.
10. Ventilate the patient and check that this is effective.
11. Secure the tube to prevent dislodgement.

Complications of cricothyroidotomy
These include:

- Asphyxia.
- Aspiration of blood or secretions.
- Haemorrhage or haematoma.
- Creation of a false passage into the tissues.
- Surgical emphysema (subcutaneous or mediastinal).
- Pulmonary barotrauma.
- Subglottic oedema or stenosis.
- Oesophageal perforation.
- Cellulitis.

VENTILATION WITHOUT INTUBATION

Mouth-to-mask ventilation

1. Apply the mask to the face, using a jaw thrust grip, with the thumbs holding the mask. If using a shaped mask, it should be the right way up in children (Figure 21.7), or upside down in infants (Figure 21.8).

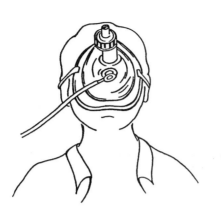

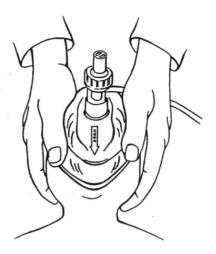

Figure 21.7. Mouth-to-mask ventilation in a child

Figure 21.8. Mouth-to-mask ventilation in an infant

2. Ensure an adequate seal.
3. Blow into the mouth port, observing the resulting chest movement.
4. Ventilate at 15–30 breaths/minute depending on the age of the child.
5. Attach oxygen to the face mask if possible.

Bag-and-mask ventilation

1. Apply the mask to the face, using a jaw thrust grip, with a thumb holding the mask (Figure 21.9).

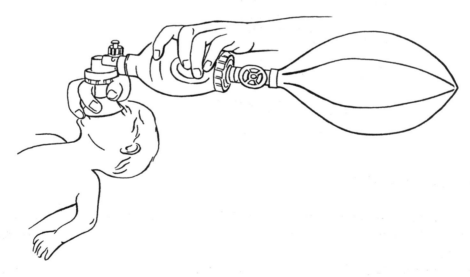

Figure 21.9. Bag-and-mask ventilation

2. Ensure an adequate seal.
3. Squeeze the bag observing the resulting chest movement.
4. Ventilate at 15–30 breaths/minute depending on the age of the child.

If a two-person technique is used, one rescuer maintains the mask seal with both hands, while the second person squeezes the self-inflating bag.

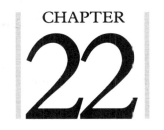

CHAPTER

22

Procedures – circulation

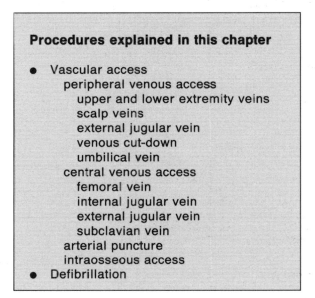

Procedures explained in this chapter

- Vascular access
  peripheral venous access
  upper and lower extremity veins
  scalp veins
  external jugular vein
  venous cut-down
  umbilical vein
  central venous access
  femoral vein
  internal jugular vein
  external jugular vein
  subclavian vein
  arterial puncture
  intraosseous access
- Defibrillation

VASCULAR ACCESS

Access to the circulation is a crucial step in delivering advanced paediatric life support. Many routes are possible; the one chosen will reflect both clinical need and the skills of the operator.

If fluids are to be given, infusion pumps or paediatric infusion sets must be used. This avoids inadvertent overtransfusion in small children.

Peripheral venous access

Upper and lower extremity veins

Veins on the dorsum of the hand, the elbow, the dorsum of the feet, and the saphenous vein at the ankle can be used for cannulation. Standard percutaneous techniques should be employed if possible.

Scalp veins

The frontal superficial, temporal posterior, auricular, supraorbital, and posterior facial veins can be used.

Equipment

- Skin cleansing swabs.
- Butterfly needle.
- Syringe and 0·9% saline.
- Short piece of tubing or bandage.

Procedure

1. Restrain the child.
2. Shave the appropriate area of the scalp.
3. Clean the skin.
4. Have an assistant distend the vein by holding a taut piece of tubing or bandaging perpendicular to it, proximal to the site of puncture.
5. Fill the syringe with 0·9% saline and flush the butterfly set.
6. Disconnect the syringe and leave the end of the tubing open.
7. Puncture the skin and enter the vein. Blood will flow back through the tubing.
8. Infuse a small quantity of fluid to see that the cannula is properly placed and then tape into position.

External jugular vein

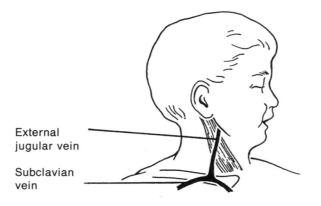

External jugular vein

Subclavian vein

Figure 22.1. The course of the external jugular vein

Equipment

- Skin cleansing swabs.
- Appropriate cannula.
- Tape.

Procedure

1. Place child in a 15–30° head-down position (or with padding under the shoulders so that the head hangs lower than the shoulders).
2. Turn the head away from the site of puncture. Restrain the child as necessary in this position.

190

3. Clean the skin over the appropriate side of the neck.
4. Identify the external jugular vein, which can be seen passing over the sternocleido-mastoid muscle at the junction of its middle and lower thirds (Figure 22.1).
5. Have an assistant place his or her finger at the lower end of the visible part of the vein just above the clavicle. This stabilises it and compresses it so that it remains distended.
6. Puncture the skin and enter the vein.
7. When free flow of blood is obtained, ensure no air bubbles are present in the tubing and then attach a giving set.
8. Tape the cannula securely in position.

Venous cut-down

If speed is essential, it may be more appropriate to use the intraosseous route for immediate access, and to cut down later for continued fluid and drug therapy.

Equipment

- Skin cleansing swabs.
- Lignocaine 1% for local anaesthetic with 2 ml syringe and 25-gauge needle.
- Scalpel.
- Curved haemostats.
- Suture and ligature material.
- Cannula.

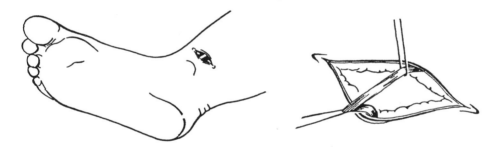

Figure 22.2. Site of long saphenous cutdown and technique

Procedure

1. Immobilise the appropriate limb.
2. Clean the skin.
3. Identify the surface landmarks for the relevant vein. These are shown in Table 22.1.

Table 22.1. Surface anatomy of the brachial and long saphenous veins

Child	Brachial	Saphenous (Figure 22.2)
Infant	One fingerbreadth lateral to the medial epicondyle of the humerus	Half a fingerbreadth superior and anterior to the medial malleolus
Small children	Two fingerbreadths lateral to the medial epicondyle of the humerus	One fingerbreadth superior and anterior to the medial malleolus
Older children	Three fingerbreadths lateral to the medial epicondyle of the humerus	Two fingerbreadths superior and anterior to the medial malleolus

4. If the child is responsive to pain, infiltrate the skin with 1% lignocaine.
5. Make an incision perpendicular to the course of the vein through the skin.
6. Using the curved haemostat tips, bluntly dissect the subcutaneous tissue.
7. Identify the vein and free 1–2 cm in length.
8. Pass a proximal and a distal ligature (Figure 22.2).
9. Tie off the distal end of the vein, keeping the ends of the tie long.
10. Make a small hole in the upper part of the exposed vein with a scalpel blade or fine-pointed scissors.
11. While holding the distal tie to stabilise the vein, insert the cannula.
12. Secure this in place with the upper ligature. Do not tie this too tightly and cause occlusion.
13. Attach a syringe filled with 0·9% saline to the cannula and ensure that fluid flows freely up the vein. If free-flow does not occur, then either the tip of the cannula is against a venous valve or the cannula may be wrongly placed in the adventitia surrounding the vein. Withdrawing the catheter will improve flow in the former case.
14. Once fluid flows freely, tie the distal ligature around the catheter to help immobilise it.
15. Close the incision site with interrupted sutures.
16. Fix the catheter or cannula to the skin and cover with a sterile dressing.

Umbilical vein

Venous access via the umbilical vein is a rapid and simple technique. It is used during newborn resuscitation.

Equipment

- Skin cleansing swabs.
- Umbilical tape.
- Scalpel.
- Syringe and 0·9% saline.
- Catheter.

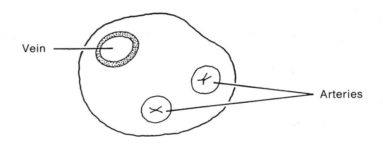

Figure 22.3. Umbilical cord cross-section

Procedure

1. Loosely tie the umbilical tape around the cord.
2. Cut the cord with a scalpel, leaving a 1 cm strip distal to the tape.
3. Identify the umbilical vein. Three vessels will be seen in the stump: two will be small and contracted (the arteries), and one will be dilated (the vein) (Figure 22.3).
4. Fill a French 5-gauge catheter with 0·9% saline.
5. Insert the catheter into the vein, and advance it approximately 5 cm.
6. Tighten the umbilical tape to secure the catheter. A purse-string suture may be used later to stitch the catheter in place.

Central venous access

Central access can be obtained through the femoral, internal jugular, external jugular, and (in older children) subclavian veins. The Seldinger technique is safe and effective. The femoral vein is often used as it is relatively easy to cannulate away from the chest during cardiopulmonary resuscitation. Central venous access via the neck veins is not without dangers, and may be difficult in emergency situations. The course of the central veins in the neck is shown in Figure 22.4.

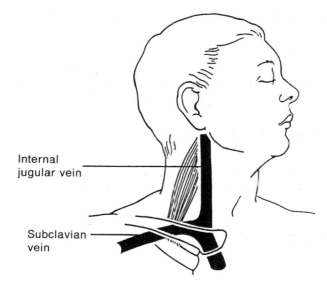

Internal
jugular vein

Subclavian
vein

Figure 22.4. The course of the central veins of the neck

Femoral vein
Equipment

- Skin cleansing swabs.
- Lignocaine 1% for local anaesthetic with 2 ml syringe and 23-gauge needle.
- Syringe and 0·9% saline.
- Seldinger cannulation set:
    syringe;
    needle;
    Seldinger guide wire;
    cannula.
- Suture material.
- Prepared paediatric infusion set.
- Tape.

Procedure

1. Place the child supine with the groin exposed and leg slightly abducted at the hip. Restrain the child's leg and body as necessary.
2. Clean the skin around the appropriate side.
3. Identify the puncture site. The femoral vein is found by palpating the femoral artery. The vein lies directly medial to the artery.
4. If the child is responsive to pain, infiltrate the area with 1% lignocaine.
5. Attach the needle to the syringe.

6. Keeping one finger on the artery to mark its position, introduce the needle at a 45° angle pointing towards the patient's head directly over the femoral vein. Keep the syringe in line with the child's leg. Advance the needle, pulling back on the plunger of the syringe all the time.
7. As soon as blood flows back into the syringe, take the syringe off the needle. Immediately occlude the end of the needle to prevent blood loss.
8. If the vein is not found withdraw the needle to the skin, locate the artery again, and advance as in (6) above.
9. Insert the Seldinger wire into the needle, and into the vein.
10. Withdraw the needle along the wire, ensuring that the wire is not dislodged from the vein.
11. Place the catheter over the wire and advance it through the skin, into the vein.
12. Suture the catheter in place.
13. Withdraw the wire, immediately occluding the end of the cannula to prevent blood loss.
14. Attach the infusion set.
15. Tape the infusion set tubing in place.

Internal jugular vein
Equipment

- Skin cleansing swabs.
- Lignocaine 1% for local anaesthetic with 2 ml syringe and 23-gauge needle.
- Syringe and 0·9% saline.
- Seldinger cannulation set:
    syringe;
    needle;
    Seldinger guide wire;
    cannula.
- Suture material.
- Prepared paediatric infusion set.
- Tape.

Procedure

1. Place the child in a 15–30° head-down position.
2. Turn the head away from the side that is to be cannulated and restrain the child as necessary.
3. Clean the skin around the appropriate side of the neck.
4. Identify the puncture site. This is found at the apex of the triangle formed by the two lower heads of the sternomastoid and the clavicle.
5. If the child is responsive to pain, infiltrate the area with 1% lignocaine.
6. Attach the needle to the syringe and puncture the skin at the appropriate place (see (4) above).
7. Direct the needle downwards at 30° to the skin; advance the needle towards the nipple, pulling back on the plunger of the syringe all the time.
8. As soon as the blood flows back into the syringe, take the syringe off the needle. Immediately occlude the end of the needle to prevent air embolism.
9. If the vein is not found withdraw the needle to the skin, and advance it again some 5–10° laterally.
10. Insert the Seldinger wire into the needle, and into the vein.
11. Withdraw the needle along the wire, ensuring that the wire is not dislodged from the vein.

12. Place the catheter over the wire and advance it through the skin, into the vein.
13. Suture the catheter in place.
14. Withdraw the wire, immediately occluding the end of the cannula to prevent air embolism.
15. Attach the infusion set.
16. Tape the infusion set tubing in place.
17. Obtain a chest radiograph in order to see the position of the catheter and to exclude pneumothorax.

External jugular vein

By using the Seldinger technique it is possible to obtain central venous access via the external jugular vein as described below. The anatomy is such that passage into the central veins can sometimes be more difficult compared to other approaches.

Equipment

- Skin cleansing swabs.
- Lignocaine 1% for local anaesthetic with 2 ml syringe and 25-gauge needle.
- Syringe and 0·9% saline.
- Seldinger cannulation set:
    syringe;
    needle;
    Seldinger guide wire (J wire);
    cannula.
- Suture material.
- Prepared paediatric infusion set.
- Tape.

Procedure

1. Place child in a 15–30° head-down position (or with padding under the shoulders so that the head hangs lower than the shoulders).
2. Turn the head away from the site of puncture. Restrain the child as necessary in this position.
3. Clean the skin over the appropriate side of the neck.
4. Identify the external jugular vein which can be seen passing over the sternocleido-mastoid muscle at the junction of its middle and lower thirds.
5. Have an assistant place his or her finger at the lower end of the visible part of the vein just above the clavicle. This stabilises it and compresses it so that it remains distended.
6. Attach the needle to the syringe and puncture the vein.
7. As soon as free-flow of blood is obtained, take off the syringe and occlude the end of the needle.
8. Insert a J wire into the needle and into the vein.
9. Advance the J wire. There may be some resistance as the wire reaches the valve at the proximal end of the vein. Gently advance and withdraw the wire until it passes this obstacle.
10. Gently advance the wire.
11. Withdraw the needle along the wire, ensuring that the wire is not dislodged from the vein.
12. Place the catheter over the wire and advance it through the skin, into the vein.
13. Suture the catheter in place.

14. Withdraw the wire, immediately occluding the end of the cannula to prevent air embolism.
15. Attach the infusion set.
16. Tape the infusion set tubing in place.
17. Obtain a chest radiograph in order to see the position of the catheter and to exclude pneumothorax.

Subclavian vein
Equipment

- Skin cleansing swabs.
- Lignocaine 1% for local anaesthetic with 2 ml syringe and 23-gauge needle.
- Syringe and 0·9% saline.
- Seldinger cannulation set:
     syringe;
     needle;
     Seldinger guide wire;
     cannula.
- Suture material.
- Prepared paediatric infusion set.
- Tape.

Procedure

1. Place the child in a 15–30° head-down position.
2. Turn the head away from the site that is to be cannulated and restrain the child as necessary.
3. Clean the skin over the upper side of the chest to the clavicle.
4. Identify the puncture site. This is 1 cm below the mid-point of the clavicle.
5. If the child is responsive to pain, infiltrate the area with 1% lignocaine.
6. Attach the needle to the syringe and puncture the skin at the appropriate place (see (4) above).
7. Direct the needle under the clavicle, "stepping down" off the bone.
8. Once under the clavicle, direct the needle towards the suprasternal notch. Advance the needle, pulling back on the plunger of the syringe all the time, and staying as superficial as possible.
9. As soon as the blood flows back into the syringe, take the syringe off the needle. Immediately occlude the end of the needle to prevent air embolism.
10. If the vein is not found, slowly withdraw the needle, continuing to pull back on the plunger. If the vein has been crossed inadvertently, free-flow will often be established during this manoeuvre.
11. If the vein is still not found repeat (7) to (10).
12. Insert the Seldinger wire into the needle, and into the vein.
13. Withdraw the needle along the wire, ensuring that the wire is not dislodged from the vein.
14. Place the catheter over the wire and advance it through the skin, into the vein.
15. Suture the catheter in place.
16. Withdraw the wire, immediately occluding the end of the cannula to prevent air embolism.
17. Attach the infusion set.
18. Tape the infusion set tubing in place.
19. Obtain a chest radiograph in order to see the position of the catheter and to exclude pneumothorax.

Arterial puncture

Arterial cannulation is used to obtain blood samples for oxygen levels and acid–base balance. In children the radial and posterior tibial arteries are the preferred sites because collateral supply is good.

Radial artery puncture
Equipment

- Skin cleansing swabs.
- Heparinised syringe.
- Butterfly needle or needle.
- Gauze, pad, and tapes.

Procedure

1. Before using the radial artery check that an ulnar artery is present and patent. Occlude both arteries at the wrist then release the pressure on the ulnar artery; the circulation should return to the hand. (It will flush pink.) If this does not happen, do not proceed with a radial puncture on that side.
2. Keep the wrist hyperextended and restrained, and palpate the radial artery.
3. Clean the skin.
4. Insert the needle over the artery at 45° to the skin and advance it slowly. When the artery is punctured blood will be seen to pulsate into the syringe.
5. Collect the required amount of blood and withdraw the needle.
6. Compress the puncture site firmly for at least 5 minutes to prevent the formation of a haematoma.
7. Ensure that there are no air bubbles in the blood sample and either send it for analysis immediately or place it on ice if any delay is anticipated.

In very small babies a 23-gauge needle can be used to puncture the artery and blood collected (into a heparinised capillary tube) from the well of the needle.

Intraosseous transfusion

The technique of intraosseous transfusion is not new. It was used in the 1930s as a quick method of gaining vascular access (the only alternatives were to use a reusable, resharpened metal needle or to perform a venous cut-down). Because it is important to achieve vascular access quickly in many life-threatening situations, intraosseous infusion is again being recommended. Specially designed needles make this quick and easy. It is indicated if other attempts at venous access fail, or if they will take longer than 2 minutes to carry out.

Equipment

- Alcohol swabs.
- An 18-gauge needle with trochar (at least 1·5 cm in length).
- A 5 ml syringe.
- A 50 ml syringe.
- Infusion fluid.

Procedure

1. Identify the infusion site. Fractured bones should be avoided, as should limbs with fractures proximal to possible sites. The landmarks for the upper tibial and lower femoral sites are shown below, and the former approach is illustrated in Figure 22.5.

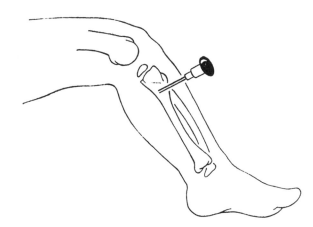

Figure 22.5. Tibial technique for intraosseous infusion

Surface anatomy for intraosseous infusions	
Tibial	*Femoral*
Anterior surface, 2–3 cm below the tibial tuberosity	Anterolateral surface, 3 cm above the lateral condyle

2. Clean the skin over the chosen site.
3. Insert the needle at 90° to the skin.
4. Continue to advance the needle until a "give" is felt as the cortex is penetrated.
5. Attach the 5 ml syringe and aspirate to confirm correct positioning.
6. Attach the filled 50 ml syringe and push in the infusion fluid in boluses.

DEFIBRILLATION

In order to achieve the optimum outcome defibrillation must be performed quickly and efficiently. This requires the following:

*   Correct paddle position.
*   Correct paddle placement.
*   Good paddle contact.
*   Correct energy selection.

Many defibrillators are available. Providers of advanced paediatric life support should make sure that they are familiar with those they may have to use.

Correct paddle selection

Most defibrillators are supplied with adult paddles attached (13 cm diameter, or equivalent area). Paddles of 4·5 cm diameter are suitable for use in infants, and ones of 8 cm diameter should be used for small children.

Correct paddle placement

The usual placement is anterolateral. One paddle is put over the apex in the mid-axillary line, and the other is placed just to the right of the sternum, immediately below the clavicle (Figure 22.6).

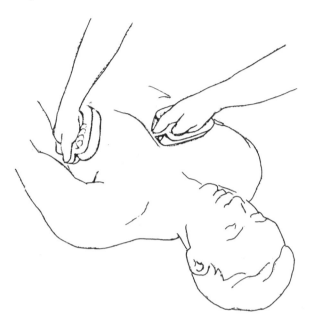

Figure 22.6. Standard anterolateral paddle placement

If the anteroposterior placement is used, one paddle is placed just to the left side of the lower part of the sternum, and the other just below the tip of the left scapula (Figure 22.7).

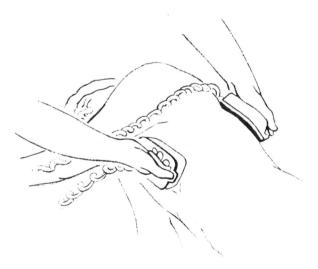

Figure 22.7. Anteroposterior paddle placement

Good paddle contact

Gel pads or electrode gel should always be used (if the latter, care should be taken not to join the two areas of application). Firm pressure should be applied to the paddles.

199

Correct energy selection

The recommended levels are shown in Chapters 6 and 10.

Safety

A defibrillator delivers enough current to *cause* cardiac arrest. The user must ensure that other rescuers are not in physical contact with the patient (or the trolley) at the moment the shock is delivered.

Procedure

Basic life support should be interrupted for the shortest possible time (6–9 below)

1. Apply gel pads or electrode gel
2. Select the correct paddles
3. Select the energy required
4. Press the charge button
5. Wait until the defibrillator is charged
6. Place the electrodes onto the pads of gel, and apply firm pressure
7. Shout "Stand back!"
8. Check that all other rescuers are clear
9. Deliver the shock

23

Procedures – trauma

Procedures explained in this chapter

- Chest decompression
    needle thoracocentesis
    chest drain placement
- Pericardiocentesis
- Femoral nerve block
- Diagnostic peritoneal lavage
- Spinal care
    cervical spine immobilisation
        application of a cervical collar
        application of sandbags and tape
    log-rolling

NEEDLE THORACOCENTESIS

This procedure can be life saving and can be performed quickly with minimum equipment. It should be followed by chest drain placement.

Minimum equipment

- Alcohol swabs.
- Large over-the-needle intravenous cannula (16-gauge or larger).
- 20 ml syringe.

Procedure

1. Identify the second intercostal space in the mid-clavicular line on the side of the pneumothorax (the *opposite* side to the direction of tracheal deviation).
2. Swab the chest wall with surgical preparation solution or an alcohol swab.
3. Attach the syringe to the cannula.

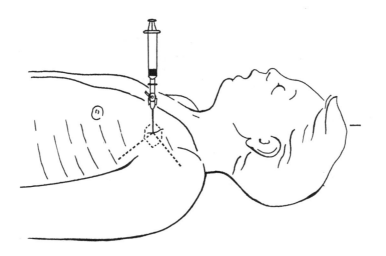

Figure 23.1. Needle thoracocentesis

4. Insert the cannula vertically into the chest wall, just above the rib below, aspirating all the time (Figure 23.1).
5. If air is aspirated remove the needle, leaving the plastic cannula in place.
6. Tape the cannula in place and proceed to chest drain insertion as soon as possible.

If needle thoracocentesis is attempted, and the patient does not have a tension pneumothorax, the chance of causing a pneumothorax is 10–20%. Patients who have had this procedure must have a chest radiograph, and will require chest drainage if ventilated.

CHEST DRAIN PLACEMENT

Chest drain placement should be performed using the open technique described here. This minimises lung damage. In general, the largest size drain that will pass between the ribs should be used.

Minimum equipment

- Skin prep and surgical drapes.
- Scalpel.
- Large clamps × 2.
- Suture.
- (Local anaesthetic.)
- Scissors.
- Chest drain tube.

Procedure

1. Decide on the insertion site (usually the fifth intercostal space in the mid-axillary line) on the side with the pneumothorax (Figure 23.2).
2. Swab the chest wall with surgical prep or an alcohol swab.

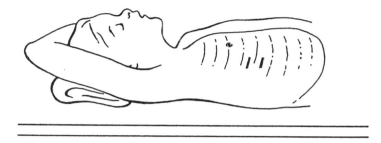

Figure 23.2. Chest drain insertion – landmarks

3. Use local anaesthetic if necessary.
4. Make a 2–3 cm skin incision along the line of the intercostal space, just above the rib below.
5. Bluntly dissect through the subcutaneous tissues just over the top of the rib below, and puncture the parietal pleura with the tip of the clamp.
6. Put a gloved finger into the incision and clear the path into the pleura (Figure 23.3).

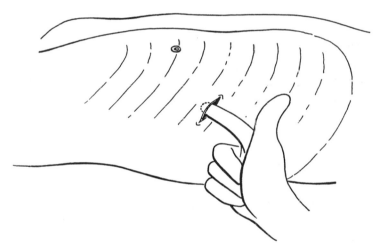

Figure 23.3. Chest drain insertion – clearing the path

7. Advance the chest drain tube into the pleural space.
8. Ensure the tube is in the pleural space by listening for air movement, and by looking for fogging of the tube during expiration.
9. Connect the chest drain tube to an underwater seal.
10. Suture the drain in place, and secure with tape.
11. Obtain a chest radiograph.

PERICARDIOCENTESIS

The removal of a small amount of fluid from the pericardial sac can be life saving. The procedure is not without risks and the ECG should be closely monitored throughout. An acute injury pattern (ST segment changes or a widened QRS) indicates ventricular damage by the needle.

Minimum equipment

- ECG monitor.
- (Local anaesthetic.)
- 20 ml syringe.
- Skin prep and surgical drapes.
- 6 inch over-the-needle cannula (16-gauge or 18-gauge).

Procedure

1. Swab the xiphoid and subxiphoid areas with surgical prep or an alcohol swab.
2. Use local anaesthetic if necessary.
3. Assess the patient for any significant mediastinal shift if possible.
4. Attach the syringe to the needle.
5. Puncture the skin 1–2 cm inferior to the left side of the xiphoid junction at a 45° angle (Figure 23.4).

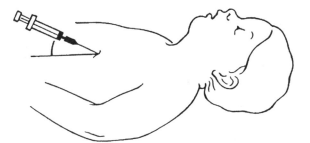

Figure 23.4. Needle pericardiocentesis – angle

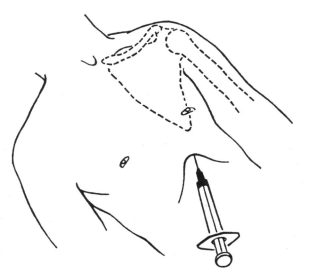

Figure 23.5. Needle pericardiocentesis – direction

6. Advance the needle towards the tip of the left scapula, aspirating all the time (Figure 23.5).
7. Watch the ECG monitor for signs of myocardial injury.
8. Once fluid is withdrawn, aspirate as much as possible (unless it is possible to withdraw limitless amounts of blood in which case a ventricle has probably been entered).
9. If the procedure is successful, remove the needle leaving the cannula in the pericardial sac. Secure in place and seal with a three-way tap. This allows later repeat aspirations should tamponade recur.

FEMORAL NERVE BLOCK

The femoral nerve supplies the femur with sensation and is useful in cases of femoral fracture. The technique may also be of benefit when analgesic agents would interfere with the management or assessment of other injuries. A long-acting local anaesthetic agent should be used so that radiographs and splinting can be undertaken with minimal distress to the child.

Equipment

- Antiseptic swabs to clean.
- Lignocaine 1%.
- A 2 ml syringe and 25-gauge needle.
- Syringe (5 or 10 ml) and 21-gauge needle.
- Bupivacaine 0·5%.

Table 23.1. Volume of bupivacaine (Marcaine) needed

Bupivacaine volume (ml)	Age (years)
10	> 12
5	5–12
1/year	< 5

Procedure

1. Move the fractured limb gently so that the femur lies in abduction and the ipsilateral groin is exposed.
2. Swab the groin clean with antiseptic solution.
3. Identify the femoral artery and keep one finger on it. The femoral nerve lies immediately lateral to the artery.
4. Using the 2 ml syringe and 25-gauge needle, infiltrate the skin just lateral to the artery. Aspirate the syringe frequently to ensure that the needle is not in a vessel.
5. Inject the bupivacaine around the nerve using the 21-gauge needle, taking care not to puncture the artery or vein.
6. Wait until anaesthesia occurs (bupivacaine may take up to 20 minutes to have its full effect).

DIAGNOSTIC PERITONEAL LAVAGE

The technique described here is designed to maximise the selectivity and specificity of diagnostic peritoneal lavage. Special care should be taken when performing diagnostic peritoneal lavage in children, otherwise the unwary operator may be caught out by the relative thinness of the abdominal wall, the intra-abdominal position of the bladder, and the high incidence of acute gastric dilatation.

Equipment

- Antiseptic solution.
- Lignocaine 1% with adrenaline.
- Scalpel.
- Self-retaining retractors.
- Suture material.
- 500 ml sterile normal (physiological) saline (warmed).
- Sterile drapes.
- Syringe and needle.
- Artery forceps.
- Scissors.
- Peritoneal lavage catheter.
- Giving set.

Procedure

1. Ensure that the urinary bladder is catheterised and drained, and that a gastric tube has been passed to decompress the stomach.
2. Surgically prepare the abdomen with antiseptic solution and drapes.
3. Identify the site for incision – one-third of the way down from the umbilicus towards the pubis in the mid-line.
4. Anaesthetise the area to the peritoneum with 1% lignocaine and adrenaline.
5. Make a vertical incision through skin and subcutaneous tissue in the mid-line.
6. Incise the fascia.
7. Ensure haemostasis.
8. Apply two clips to the peritoneum and gently lift it away from underlying structures.
9. Using the scissors cut between the two clips – making a small hole in the peritoneum.
10. Insert the dialysis catheter through the hole, and gently advance it caudally into the pelvis.
11. Connect the dialysis catheter to a syringe and aspirate.
12. If blood is not aspirated, connect the catheter to the giving set and infuse 10 ml/kg of the warmed saline.
13. Remove any remaining saline from the bag.
14. If the patient is stable leave this fluid for 5–10 minutes, and then allow it to syphon out by placing the bag on the floor. This may take some time (30 minutes or more).
15. Send a sample of fluid to the laboratory for analysis.
16. Remove the catheter and close the wound in layers.

CERVICAL SPINE IMMOBILISATION

All children with serious trauma must be treated as though they have a cervical spine injury. It is only when adequate investigations have been performed and a neuro-surgical or orthopaedic consultation obtained, if necessary, that the decision to remove cervical spine protection should be taken. In-line cervical stabilisation should be applied until a hard collar has been applied, and sandbags and tape are in position as described below.

Two techniques are described. It is necessary to apply both to achieve adequate cervical spine control.

206

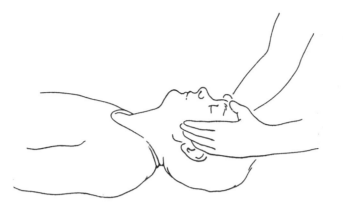

Figure 23.6. In-line cervical stabilisation

Application of a cervical collar

The key to successful, effective, collar application lies in selecting the correct size.

Minimum equipment
- Measuring device.
- Range of paediatric hard collars.

Method
1. Ensure in-line cervical stabilisation is maintained throughout by a second person.
2. Using the manufacturer's method, select a correctly sized collar.
3. Fully unfold and assemble the collar.
4. Taking care not to cause movement, pass the flat part of the collar behind the neck.
5. Fold the shaped part of the collar round and place it under the child's chin.
6. Fold the flat part of the collar with its integral joining device (usually Velcro tape) around until it meets the shaped part.
7. Reassess the correct fit of the collar.
8. If the fit is wrong, slip the flat part of the collar out from behind the neck, taking care not to cause movement. Select the correct size and recommence the procedure.
9. If the fit is correct secure the joining device.
10. Ensure that in-line cervical stabilisation is maintained until sandbags and tape are in position.

Sandbags and tape

Equipment
- Two sandbags.
- Strong narrow tape.

Method
1. Ensure in-line cervical stabilisation is maintained by a second person throughout.
2. Place a sandbag either side of the head.
3. Apply tape across the forehead and securely attach it to the long spinal board or trolley.
4. Apply tape across the chin piece of the hard collar and securely attach it to the long spinal board or trolley.

Exceptions

Two groups of children cause particular difficulty. The first (and most common) is the frightened, uncooperative child; the second is the child who is hypoxic and combative. In both cases, overzealous immobilisation of the head and neck may paradoxically increase cervical spine movement. This is because these children will fight to escape from any restraint. In such cases a hard collar should be applied, and no attempt made to immobilise the head with sandbags and tape.

LOG-ROLLING

In order to minimise the chances of exacerbating unrecognised spinal cord injury, non-essential movements of the spine must be avoided until adequate examination and investigations have excluded it. If manoeuvres that might cause spinal movement are essential (for example, during examination of the back in the course of the secondary survey) then log-rolling should be performed. The aim of log-rolling is to maintain the orientation of the spine during turning of the child. The basic requirements are an adequate number of carers and good control.

Method

1. Gather together enough staff to roll the child. In larger children four people will be required; three will be required in smaller children and infants.
2. Place the staff as shown in Table 23.2.
3. Ensure each member of staff knows what they are going to do as shown in Table 23.3.
4. Carry out essential manoeuvres as quickly as possible.

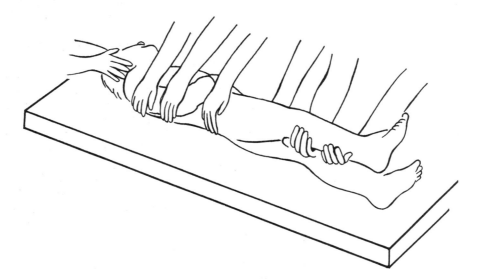

Figure 23.7.   Log-rolling a child (four-person technique)

Table 23.2. Position of staff in log-rolling

Staff member no.	Position of staff for	
	Smaller child and infant	Larger child
1	Head	Head
2	Chest	Chest
3	Legs and pelvis	Pelvis
4		Legs

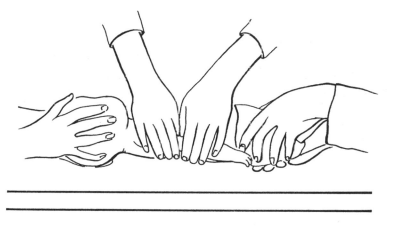

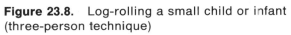

Figure 23.8. Log-rolling a small child or infant (three-person technique)

Table 23.3. Tasks of individual members of staff

Staff member – position	Task
Head	Hold either side of the head (as for in-line cervical stabilisation), and maintain the orientation of the head with the body in all planes during turning *Control the log-roll by telling other staff when to roll and when to lay the child back onto the trolley*
Chest	Reach over the child and carefully place both hands under the chest. When told to roll the child support the weight of the chest, and maintain stability. Watch the movement of the head at all times and roll the chest at the same rate
Pelvis and legs	*This only applies to smaller children and infants. If it is not possible to control the pelvis and legs at the same time get additional help immediately* Place one hand either side of the pelvis over the iliac crests. Cradle the child's legs between the forearms. When told to roll the child, grip the pelvis and legs and move them together. Watch the movement of the head and chest at all times, and roll the pelvis and legs at the same rate
Pelvis	Place one hand either side of the pelvis over the iliac crests. When told to roll the child, grip the pelvis and roll it. Watch the movement of the head and chest at all times and roll the pelvis at the same rate
Legs	Support the weight of the far leg by placing both hands under it. When told to roll the child watch the movement of the chest and pelvis and roll the leg at the same rate

CHAPTER
24

Transport of children

Sick or injured children may initially be taken to a unit that can offer adequate resuscitation or stabilisation, but is unable to offer further acute or long-term medical management. Such children must be transported to another hospital or department. Reviews of children transferred to neurosurgical units for tertiary care have revealed several potentially avoidable factors which have contributed to death or increased morbidity. One of these is failure to recognise the extent of injury, especially the presence of splenic or hepatic injury. Others are lack of adequate preparation for transport, and lack of suitable support during the journey between hospitals.

It is essential to evaluate, resuscitate, and stabilise a child's condition before moving him or her. Whatever the injury or illness the airway must be secured and ventilation must be adequate. Intravenous access must be established and fluids and/or life-saving drugs given. Proper evaluation requires a thorough examination to show whether any orthopaedic, surgical, or medical procedures should be carried out prior to transportation. Baseline haematological and biochemical samples should be taken when the intravenous lines are placed and essential radiographs should be carried out at this time.

The staff at the receiving hospital or department must be contacted prior to arranging transport. They must be clearly told what has happened, the state of the child, the treatment received, and what transport facilities and staff are needed. Both teams can then decide if the child is stable enough for transport, and whether the referring or receiving hospital will provide the staff to supervise the transfer.

It should be calculated that the journey will take twice as long as the time calculated for it will take. Traffic jams or weather conditions may lead to unavoidable delays. It is important to carry adequate stocks of fluids, drugs, and oxygen. For very long journeys, pick-up points for oxygen should be prearranged prior to departure.

The child's notes, radiographs, charts, and any cross-matched blood should be taken to the receiving unit. Results of investigations that become available after the child has left should be communicated to the receiving unit immediately.

Parents must be kept fully informed of the situation. If clear explanations are given as to why and where a child is being taken it lessens their anxiety and increases their cooperation.

> **Checklist prior to transporting a child**
>
> - Is the airway protected and ventilation satisfactory? (Substantiated by blood gases, pH and pulse oximetry.)
> - Is the neck properly immobilised?
> - Is there sufficient oxygen available for the journey?
> - Is vascular access *secure* and will the pumps in use during transport work by battery?
> - Have adequate fluids been given prior to transport?
> - Are fractured limbs appropriately splinted and immobilised?
> - Are appropriate monitors in use?
> - Will the child be sufficiently warm during the journey?
> - Is all documentation available? Include:
>   child's name;
>   age;
>   date of birth;
>   weight;
>   radiographs taken;
>   clinical notes;
>   observation charts;
>   neurological observation chart;
>   the time and route of all drugs given;
>   fluid charts;
>   ventilation records;
>   results of investigations.
> - Has the case been discussed with the receiving team directly?
> - Have plans been discussed with the parents?

PAEDIATRIC TRANSFER EQUIPMENT

Airway

1. Oropharyngeal airway sizes 000, 00, 0, 1, 2, 3.
2. Endotracheal tubes sizes 2·5–7·5 mm uncuffed (in 0·5 mm steps) and 7·5 mm cuffed.
3. Laryngoscopes:
    (a) straight paediatric blade;
    (b) adult curved blade.
4. Magill's forceps.
5. Yankauer's sucker.
6. Soft suction catheters.
7. Needle cricothyroidotomy set.

Breathing

1. Oxygen masks with reservoir.
2. Self-inflating bags (with reservoir):
    (a) 240 ml infant size;
    (b) 500 ml child size;
    (c) 1600 ml adult size.
3. Face masks:
    (a) infant – circular 01, 1, 2;
    (b) child – anatomical 2, 3;
    (c) adult – anatomical 4, 5.
4. Catheter mount and connectors.
5. Ayre's T-piece.

Circulation

1. ECG monitor – defibrillator (with paediatric paddles).
2. Non-invasive blood pressure monitor (with infant- and child-sized cuffs).
3. Pulse oximeter (with infant- and child-sized probes).
4. Intravenous access requirements:
   (a) intravenous cannulae (as available): 18–25 gauge;
   (b) intraosseous infusion needles: 16–18 gauge;
   (c) graduated burette;
   (d) intravenous giving sets;
   (e) syringes: 1–50 ml.
5. Intravenous drip monitoring device.
6. Cut-down set.

Fluids

- Saline 0·9%.
- Hartmann's solution or Ringer's lactate.
- Dextrose 4% and 0·18% saline.
- Dextrose 5%.
- Colloid.
- Plasma.

Drugs

- Adrenaline 1:10 000.
- Atropine 1 mg in 10 ml.
- Sodium bicarbonate 8·4%.
- Dopamine 40 mg/ml.
- Lignocaine 1%.
- Dextrose 10%, 25%, and 50%.
- Calcium chloride 10%.
- Frusemide 10 mg/ml.
- Mannitol 10% or 20%.
- Antibiotics – penicillin, chloramphenicol, gentamicin, ampicillin, ceftazidime, cefotaxime.

Miscellaneous

- Stick test for glucose.
- Chest drain set.

A

Acid–base balance

ACIDOSIS

Acidosis is a common problem in sick children. Under normal circumstances the blood pH is tightly controlled between 7·35 and 7·45. Although this sounds like very little variation, it has to be remembered that there is a logarithmic relationship between pH and hydrogen ion concentration ($[H^+]$). Thus a pH rise from 7·35 to 7·45 represents a fall in $[H^+]$ from 45 to 35 nmol/l. When the pH falls significantly from normal values to 7·1 the $[H^+]$ has doubled to 80 nmol/l. Many buffers exist to protect against the pH changes that occur as H^+ production increases in sepsis, injury, poor perfusion, and catabolism, or if there is failure to excrete normal acids produced.

It is easy to get confused by the complexities of the interrelationships between buffering systems (red blood cells, plasma proteins, and bicarbonate). Similarly, understanding the relationship between pH, bicarbonate, and $P\text{CO}_2$ within the Henderson–Hasselbach equation often causes dismay. The practical management of a patient with acidosis can be simplified by the application of straightforward rules.

Acidosis is the result of an insult, and correction will occur if the original insult is dealt with. Practical intervention to maintain the circulation and relieve shock will also improve acidosis because plasma and blood are buffering agents. With normal renal function and bicarbonate production, most acidoses will then correct themselves in time. Thus intervention is only required if the pH has fallen so low that it has an effect on the ability of the cells to function normally. This level is arbitrary, but is taken as a pH below 7·15. When the pH is down at this level the reason must be sought.

Bicarbonate mops up hydrogen ions to produce CO_2 and water:

$$H^+ + HCO_3^- \rightleftharpoons H_2O + CO_2$$

These four substances are in balance. Thus increased removal of CO_2 will remove hydrogen ions and improve acidosis in the short term (at the expense of the serum bicarbonate). Retention of CO_2 will lead to a worsening of acidosis by preventing incorporation of hydrogen ions into water, at least until bicarbonate production is increased to provide extra buffer. Acidosis in the face of a low or normal CO_2 is thus metabolic in origin and is due to increased production of or failure to excrete hydrogen ions. Acidosis in the face of a high CO_2 is respiratory. Often a mixed picture occurs.

Figure A.1 shows the relationship between pH and bicarbonate concentration at different levels of CO_2. It can be seen that at a given bicarbonate concentration the pH falls as the CO_2 rises. Also it can be seen that at lower pH levels small falls in bicarbonate concentration produce dramatic reductions in pH. Similarly, at low pH values small amounts of bicarbonate cause large shifts in pH. The nearer the pH gets to normal the larger the amount of bicarbonate needed to improve the correction.

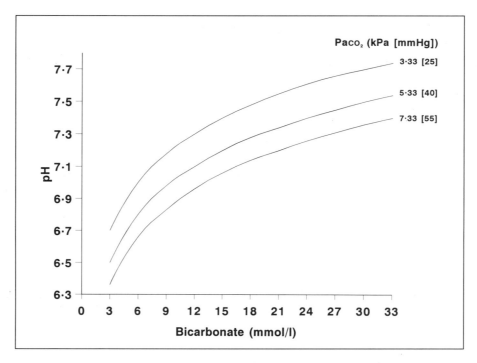

Figure A.1. The relationship between pH, bicarbonate, and carbon dioxide

In a clinical situation, complex calculations of the amount of bicarbonate needed are unnecessary. As correction is only going to be attempted at a pH of below 7·15 then a single dose of 2·5 mmol/kg (2·5 ml/kg of 8·4% $NaHCO_3$) should be given. This is based on the knowledge that bicarbonate will quickly be distributed between the extracellular and intracellular fluids (which total about 600 ml/kg). Thus a dose of 2·5 mmol/kg will raise the serum bicarbonate by just over 4 mmol/l. Re-examination of Figure A.1 shows that this rise in serum bicarbonate will usually take the pH to above 7·15. If the pH is rechecked after this dose has been given, and significant correction has not occurred, then it is either because of the presence of a high acid load or because of high acid production rates. The dose should be repeated. When correcting acidosis the serum calcium should always be checked because, in patients with severe sepsis or renal failure, hypocalcaemia can be marked and will be exacerbated by correction of acidosis which reduces the ionised calcium further. It should be remembered that correction of acidosis causes a fall in the serum potassium via intracellular movement. Thus, in patients with a low serum potassium, supplements will be required.

ALKALOSIS

Alkalosis is a much rarer problem, the two major causes being hyperventilation and vomiting.

Hyperventilation can be a manifestation of either an acute or an acute-on-chronic psychological problem. The CO_2 can fall quite low causing a significant rise in pH which is often enough to produce hypocalcaemic tetany. Use of a rebreathing bag is an excellent initial treatment. The underlying problem must then be investigated. Although psychological causes are the most common, early aspirin poisoning may cause hyperventilation and salicylate levels should be measured if this is possible.

Severe vomiting causes alkalosis in two ways. First there is direct loss of acid from the stomach. Second, and often most important, severe hypovolaemia may be induced by chronic vomiting. This causes hyperaldosteronism in an attempt to promote salt and water retention which, in turn, leads to increased renal potassium and hydrogen ion loss with bicarbonate retention. This exacerbates the alkalosis. Volume expansion with normal (physiological) saline promotes correction. Congenital hypertrophic pyloric stenosis is a good example of this physiological process in action.

ANALYSIS OF AN ARTERIAL BLOOD GAS (ABG)

The proper interpretation of an ABG sample requires clinical history, examination, knowledge of treatments given, and other laboratory investigations. In emergencies, when much of the data is lacking, interpret the findings with caution.

What is the pH? (normal 7·36–7·44)

Is there an acidosis or alkalosis? If the pH is near normal it may be due to respiratory or metabolic compensation. This compensation is never complete.

What is the $PaCO_2$? (normal 4·7–6·0 kPa, 35–45 mmHg)

This is a good indicator of ventilatory adequacy because it is inversely proportional to alveolar minute volume (respiratory rate × alveolar tidal volume). When the pH is known, it can be used to determine whether there are compensatory ventilatory changes.

What is the base excess? (normal 0–2 mmol/l)

A positive base excess indicates a metabolic alkalosis. A negative base excess indicates a metabolic acidosis. However, a mild acidosis is of benefit as it facilitates the release of oxygen from the haemoglobin molecules to tissues. For this reason a negative base excess is only treated if it is more negative than − 6 and the pH is low.

Bicarbonate and base excess are *calculated* by blood gas analysers using the Henderson–Hasselbach equation. These results must always be interpreted cautiously in clinical situations.

What is the PaO_2? (normal 10·6 kPa, > 80 mmHg in air)

The partial pressure of oxygen in the arterial blood sample must be interpreted in the light of the inspired oxygen concentration. Atmospheric pressure is approximately 100 kPa; therefore 1% is about 1 kPa.

For example, inspiring 30% O_2 from an oxygen mask would give an alveolar concentration of 20–25·5 kPa. There is a fall of about 7·5 kPa between the PO_2 at the mouth and in the alveoli.

Precautions when taking an arterial blood sample

How to take an arterial blood sample is described in Chapter 22. Certain errors must be avoided:

- Ensure an adequate sample; avoid bubbles – dead space in the syringe will allow carbon dioxide and oxygen to diffuse in or out of the sample. Seal the syringe with a plastic cap for the same reasons.
- Avoid excess heparin. Fill the dead space of a 2 ml syringe and attached needle with heparin (1000 units/ml). A pre-heparinised syringe is preferable.
- Minimise metabolism in the sample. Delay in analysis allows both oxygen consumption and carbon dioxide generation to continue in the syringe. If a delay of more than a few minutes is anticipated, store the sample on ice.

B

Fluid and electrolyte management

Fluid and electrolyte management is an essential part of both the immediate and the ongoing care of all sick children. In this appendix we will look at the following:

1. Normal requirements.
2. Dehydration.
3. Diabetic ketoacidosis.
4. Hypervolaemia.
5. Specific electrolyte problems.

NORMAL REQUIREMENTS

Volume

Blood volume is about 100 ml/kg at birth falling to about 80 ml/kg at 1 year. Total body water varies from just under 800 ml/kg in the neonate to about 600 ml/kg at 1 year; after this it varies little. Of this about two-thirds (400 ml/kg) are intracellular fluid; the rest is extracellular fluid. Thus initial expansion of vascular volume in shock can be achieved with relatively small volumes of fluid: 20 ml/kg will usually suffice. However, this volume is only a fraction of that required to correct dehydration if the fluid has been lost from all body compartments. In fact, 20 ml/kg is 2% of body weight. Clinically, dehydration, which is distributed across the fluid compartments rather than being restricted to the vascular compartment, is not detectable until it is greater than 5% (50 ml/kg).

Much is spoken about normal fluid requirements, although in truth there is no such thing. We are all aware as adults that if we drink little we do not get dehydrated and if we drink lots we merely diurese. Healthy children's kidneys are just as capable of maintaining fluid balance. Fluids in neonates are often prescribed on the basis of 150 ml/kg/day, but this is not related to fluid needs and is merely the volume of standard formula milk required to give an adequate protein and calorie intake. What is required clinically is a simple means of prescribing fluid such that patients are maintained in a well-hydrated state and passing reasonable quantities of urine. This formula then has to be modifiable in order to take account of the need for rehydration of dry patients and prevention of overhydration in patients in whom either renal function is impaired or fluid restriction is indicated (e.g. meningitis, cerebral oedema). Fluid requirement can be divided into four types:

1. For replacement of *insensible losses* through sweat, respiration, gastrointestinal loss, etc.
2. For replacement of *essential urine output*, the minimal urine output that allows excretion of urea, etc.
3. Extra fluid to maintain a *modest state of diuresis*.
4. Fluid to replace *abnormal losses* such as blood loss, severe diarrhoea, diabetic polyuria losses, etc.

A formula for calculating this fluid requirement is given in Table B.1. It is useful because it is simple, can be applied to all age ranges and is easily subdivided. The formula gives total fluid requirements, i.e. types $(1)+(2)+(3)$ above. Of this total *one-fifth* represents insensible losses, the *second fifth* represents essential urine output, and the last *three-fifths* represent extra fluid to maintain urine output. Thus this formula is easily adaptable to all states of hydration (Table B.2).

Table B.1. Normal fluid requirements

Body weight	Fluid requirement per day (ml/kg)	Fluid requirement per hour (ml/kg)
First 10 kg	100	4
Second 10 kg	50	2
Subsequent kilogram	20	1

Table B.2. Subdivisions of total fluids

Fraction of total fluid	Function	Amount given	Type of hydration
First fifth	Insensible loss	One-fifth	Insensible losses only
Second fifth	Essential urine output	Two-fifths	Severe fluid restriction
Last three-fifths	Maintenance of urine output	Three-fifths	Moderate fluid restriction
		Four- or five-fifths	Adequate fluids
		Six- to ten-fifths	Induced diuresis

For the very sick and those with renal impairment, a combination of insensible losses plus urine output, given on an hourly basis, is often the best method of fluid management.

Electrolytes

To speak of normal electrolyte requirements is as artificial as speaking of normal fluid requirements. There are obligatory losses of electrolytes in stools, urine, and sweat, and these require replacement. Any excess is simply excreted in the urine. Table B.3 shows the electrolyte content of various body fluids and Table B.4 gives electrolyte "requirements" if there are not excessive losses from any compartment. In truth these "requirements" represent quantities that, if given, maintain homoeostasis without recourse to the various hormonal and renal tubular mechanisms for maintaining the extracellular fluid composition.

Table B.3. Electrolyte contents of body fluids

Fluid	Na$^+$ (mmol/l)	K$^+$ (mmol/l)	Cl$^-$ (mmol/l)	HCO$_3^-$ (mmol/l)
Plasma	135–141	3·5–5·5	100–105	24–28
Gastric	20–80	5–20	100–150	0
Intestinal	100–140	5–15	90–130	15–65
Diarrhoea	7–96	34–150	17–164	0–75
Sweat	<70	6–15	<70	0–10

Table B.4. Normal water, electrolyte, energy, and protein requirements

Body weight	Water (ml/kg/day)	Sodium (mmol/kg/day)	Potassium (mmol/kg/day)	Energy (kcal/day)	Protein (g/day)
First 10 kg	100	2–4	1·5–2·5	110	3·00
Second 10 kg	50	1–2	0·5–1·5	75	1·50
Subsequent kilogram	20	0·5–1	0·2–0·7	30	0·75

Tables B.5 and B.6 show commonly available intravenous fluids with their composition. Their usage is described in the appropriate sections below. The main point to note is the need for precise prescription. It is clear that "dextrose saline" can refer to any one of several different preparations.

Table B.5. Commonly available crystalloid fluids

Fluid	Na$^+$ (mmol/l)	K$^+$ (mmol/l)	Cl$^-$ (mmol/l)	Energy (kcal/l)	Other
Isotonic crystalloid fluids					
Saline 0·9%	150	0	150	0	0
Saline 0·45%, dextrose 2·5%	75	0	75	100	0
Saline 0·18%, dextrose 4%	30	0	30	160	0
Dextrose 5%	0	0	0	200	0
Saline 0·18%, dextrose 4%, 10 mmol KCl/500 ml	30	20	50	160	0
Hartmann's solution Ringer's solution	131	5	111	0	Lactate
Hypertonic crystalloid solutions					
Saline 0·45%, dextrose 5%	75	0	75	200	0
Dextrose 10%	0	0	0	400	0
Saline 0·18%, dextrose 10%	30	0	30	400	0
Dextrose 20%	0	0	0	800	0

Table B.6. Commonly available colloid fluids

Colloid solutions	Na$^+$ (mmol/l)	K$^+$ (mmol/l)	Ca^{2+} (mmol/l)	Duration of actions (hours)	Comments
Albumin 4·5%	150	1	0	6	Protein buffers H$^+$
Gelofusine	154	<1	<1	3	Gelatin
Haemaccel	145	5	12·5	3	Gelatin
Pentastarch	154	0	0	7	Hydroxyethyl starch

DEHYDRATION

Dehydration is the result of abnormal fluid losses from the body which are greater than the amount that the kidneys can compensate for. The natural mechanisms for compensation have the primary aim of maintaining circulating volume and blood pressure at all cost (Figure B.1). Thus most patients with dehydration maintain their central circulation satisfactorily. Loss of central circulatory homoeostasis constitutes *hypovolaemic shock* and is dealt with in Chapter 9.

The major causes of dehydration in children are gastrointestinal disorders and diabetic ketoacidosis. Some renal disorders (polyuric tubulopathy with urinary tract infection, polyuric chronic renal failure, and diabetes insipidus) might also present in this way. Depending on the source of fluid losses and the quantities of electrolytes lost (Table B.3), dehydration can be divided into three types:

1. Isotonic dehydration.
2. Hyponatraemic dehydration.
3. Hypernatraemic dehydration.

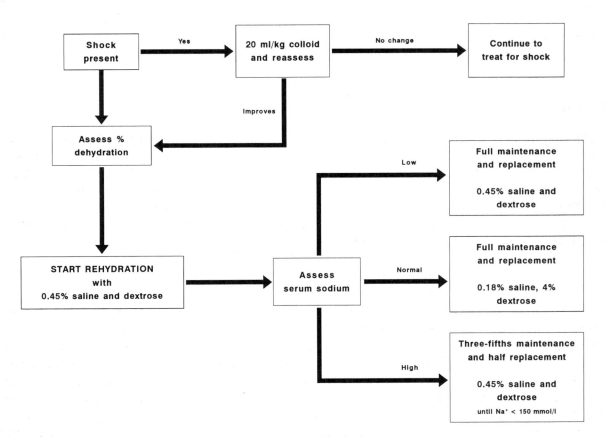

Figure B.1. Algorithm for the management of dehydration in the first 24 hours

In all three types there is a total body deficit of salt and water. Between the three types the relative amounts of salt and water loss vary. Table B.7 shows the symptoms and signs of dehydration and gives a guide towards the assessment of the degree of dehydration. On the whole, the more severe the dehydration the more probable that hypovolaemia is going to be a problem; most patients with more than 10% dehydration are hypovolaemic at presentation. However, speed of fluid loss is important. Slow, prolonged losses can give rise to massive dehydration without hypovolaemia; similarly acute, severe loss can present as hypovolaemia without apparent significant dehydration. The latter is not infrequently the case in acute gastroenteritis in infants, where acute fluid loss into the bowel causes hypovolaemia and the patient can present even before any diarrhoea has occurred.

Table B.7. Symptoms and signs of dehydration

Signs/Symptoms	Mild <5%	Moderate 5–10%	Severe >10%	Notes/Caveats
Decreased urine output	+	+	+	Beware watery diarrhoea
Dry mouth	+/−	+	+	Mouth breathers are always dry
Decreased skin turgor	−	+/−	+	Beware the thin Use several sites
Sunken anterior fontanelle	−	+	+	Crying increases pressure
Sunken eyes	−	+	+	
Decreased eyeball turgor	−	+/−	+	Difficult to assess in young
Tachypnoea	−	+/−	+	Metabolic acidosis and pyrexia worsen this
Tachycardia	−	+/−	+	Hypovolaemia, pyrexia, and irritability cause this
Drowsiness/irritability	−	+/−	+	

Management of dehydration

Mild dehydration (<5%) can often be managed with oral fluids as long as vomiting is not a major problem. It can be seen from Table B.5 that 0·18% saline, 4% dextrose gives maintenance amounts of sodium and water. Natural renal homoeostatic mechanisms will cause sodium and water retention, so the use of maintenance fluids in normal quantities is sufficient – the deficits will be corrected through an initial lower urine output.

Once the deficit exceeds 5% it is most appropriate to replace this. The deficit is calculated using the following formula:

$$\text{Percentage dehydration} \times \text{Weight (in kg)}$$

Thus a 10 kg infant who is 7·5% dehydrated requires the replacement of 750 ml. In all types of dehydration, the deficit is mainly extracellular fluid loss and ought to be replaced as normal (physiological) (0·9%) saline. If not, dilutional hyponatraemia will occur. In the absence of the need for immediate circulatory support, this replacement ought to take place over 24 hours to prevent rapid fluid shifts. In addition to the replacement of the deficit, normal maintenance fluids with 0·18% saline, 4% dextrose ought to be given. In practice, in both isotonic and hyponatraemic dehydration, it is often easiest to give the first 24-hour total fluid (deficit + maintenance) as 0·45% saline with dextrose. Following this, isotonic dehydration therapy can be continued with 0·18% saline, 4% dextrose. In hyponatraemic states continuation of 0·45% saline with dextrose will usually correct the sodium deficit easily. All fluids will require potassium. In the knowledge that significant hypokalaemia does not occur until considerable total body potassium depletion has occurred, this usually means giving twice the normal maintenance quantities, i.e. 20 mmol/500 ml.

In hypernatraemic dehydration there is a greater degree of water loss than salt loss. This leads to a higher serum osmolality, dragging fluid from the intracellular to the extracellular space, and maintaining the circulation. Thus the total fluid deficit is often higher than one would predict clinically, and there is a total body sodium deficit. The deficit ought, as before, to be replaced with normal (physiological) saline and maintenance given with 0·18% saline, 4% dextrose. Again, this can be simplified to initially just giving 0·45% saline. The risk of hypernatraemic dehydration is that over-rapid reduction in the serum sodium will lead to rapid shifts of water into the cells leading to cerebral oedema and convulsions. This can be averted by slowing down the rate of rehydration and replacing the deficit over 48 hours, giving maintenance at three-fifths the normal total. After the first 48 hours, the fluid can be changed to 0·18% saline, 4% dextrose, and once the serum sodium is below 150 mmol/l the rate of administration can be increased to normal.

The very sick child

In the very sick it cannot be assumed that normal homoeostatic mechanisms will work. The patient may be progressing into renal failure and be oliguric or inappropriately polyuric. In such cases the best management is to:

- Catheterise the patient.
- Calculate and replace the deficit, over 24 hours, with normal (physiological) saline.
- Calculate insensible losses and replace with 0·18% saline, 4% dextrose.
- Measure urine output and replace ml for ml on an hourly basis with 0·18% or 0·45% saline with dextrose, according to the type of dehydration.

This technique is applicable to all patients with all conditions in all states of hydration. Moreover, subsequent measurement of urinary electrolytes can allow exact tailoring of intravenous fluids to maintain normal serum electrolytes.

DIABETIC KETOACIDOSIS

Diabetic ketoacidosis is a special case in which a relative or absolute lack of insulin leads to an inability to metabolise glucose. This leads to hyperglycaemia and an osmotic diuresis. Once urine output exceeds the ability of the patient to drink, dehydration occurs. In addition, without insulin, fat is used as a source of energy leading to the production of large quantities of ketones and metabolic acidosis. The latter is initially compensated for by hyperventilation and a respiratory alkalosis but, as the condition progresses, the combination of acidosis, hyperosmolality, and dehydration leads to coma. Diabetic ketoacidosis is often the first presentation of diabetes, but may be a problem in known diabetics who have decompensated through illness, infection, or non-adherence to their treatment regimens.

History

The history is usually of weight loss, abdominal pain, vomiting, polyuria, and polydipsia.

Examination

Children are usually severely dehydrated with deep and rapid (Kussmaul's) respiration. They have the fruity smell of ketones on their breath. Salicylate poisoning and uraemia are differential diagnoses to be excluded. Infection often precipitates decompensation in both new and known diabetics, and must be sought.

226

Management

Assess   *A*irway
                                *B*reathing
                                *C*irculation

Give 100% oxygen. Place on a cardiac monitor (hypokalaemia can cause dysrhythmias).

Site an intravenous drip and begin fluid replacement. If shock is present, treat as discussed in Chapter 9.

Take blood for:

- Glucose.
- Urea and electrolytes, creatinine, Ca^{2+}, PO_4^{3-}.
- Full blood count and differential white cell count.
- Culture.
- Blood gases.

Take urine for:

- Culture.
- Sugar.
- Ketones.

Fluids

The principles of fluid management outlined above work as well for diabetic ketoacidosis as for any other cause of dehydration. However, as there is hyperglycaemia it is best not to give dextrose initially. Thus, having calculated deficit, maintenance, and 24-hour requirement, this can initially be given all as normal (physiological) saline, switching to 0·45% saline or 0·18% saline with dextrose once the blood sugar has fallen. With the osmotic diuresis, which will persist until the blood sugar falls, calculated fluid requirements will be an underestimate. However, this is beneficial as over-rapid rehydration is likely to cause cerebral oedema.

Insulin

Insulin ought to be given by continuous infusion. The initial dose is 0·1 unit/kg/h. Once the blood sugar falls to less than 10 mmol/l, glucose must be added to the intravenous drip. *Do not stop using insulin. This is the child's prime requirement.* Administer the insulin by separate line. Add 50 units of soluble insulin to 50 ml saline. This solution is 1 unit/ml (0·1 unit/kg/hour is equal to 0·1 × weight in kg, as ml/hour). Thus a 20 kg child would have 2 ml/hour, a 35 kg child 3·5 ml/hour. This often needs decreasing to 0·05 unit/kg/hour when blood sugar starts to fall. In a very young diabetic (under 5 years) start with the smaller dose.

Acidosis

The acidosis of diabetic ketoacidosis is initially compensated for by hyperventilation. Once the blood pH falls below 7·1, CNS depression can occur and this can prevent compensation. Almost always acidosis will correct with correction of fluid balance and cessation of ketosis with insulin therapy. Bicarbonate should be avoided unless the blood

227

pH is less than 7·0, or less than 7·1 and not improving after the first few hours of fluid and insulin therapy. Many formulae exist relating the base excess to the child's weight and the bicarbonate requirement. However, because of the logarithmic relationship between $[H^+]$ and pH (see Figure A.1), a dose of 2·5 ml/kg of 8·4% $NaHCO_3$ will correct the pH to 7·2 or 7·3 in all cases. This should be administered slowly over 2 hours by infusion. Re-check the pH after the first hour and stop the infusion if the pH is above 7·15 as the rest will correct naturally.

Other treatments

A nasogastric tube is essential as acute gastric dilatation is a common complication. Depending on the level of consciousness, bladder catheterisation may be required. Antibiotics may be indicated.

Monitoring progress

Use a flow sheet to record vital signs, neurological status, input and output of fluids, blood results, and insulin infusion rates. Record urine ketones and glucose. Initially, while intravenous insulin is in use, check blood sugar, biochemistry, and acid–base status 2-hourly.

Complications

Major complications	
Cerebral oedema	Prevent by slow normalisation of sugar and hydration; monitor neurological status hourly; treat cerebral oedema with hyperventilation and mannitol (see Chapter 12)
Hypokalaemia Cardiac dysrhythmias	Usually secondary to electrolyte disturbances
Acute renal failure	Uncommon

Any of the complications in the box requires intensive monitoring on an intensive care unit.

HYPERVOLAEMIA

Hypervolaemia and fluid overload in children is a rarer problem than dehydration. The causes tend to be either cardiac failure or renal failure. Occasionally water intoxication following deliberate ingestion or misuse of desmopressin (DDAVP) occurs.

Fluid overload from renal failure presents with raised venous pressure, a triple rhythm, and pulmonary crepitations or crackles, and is treated initially with diuretics. They may be ineffective and treatment will then require the use of oxygen, vasodilators, and urgent dialysis.

Water intoxication will usually present as convulsions secondary to cerebral oedema and hyponatraemia. Treatment is along the usual lines for patients with convulsions and coma (see Chapters 11 and 12). Severe fluid restriction will be necessary, and if hyponatraemia is severe (<120 mmol/l), fluids ought to be given as 0·9% saline. Diuretics, particularly mannitol, which causes a free water diuresis and reduces cerebral oedema, are sometimes of value.

Mild oedema may occur in any of these conditions; severe oedema does not and, when present, is usually a manifestation of nephrotic syndrome. This is important as patients with nephrotic syndrome are intravascularly fluid depleted and diuretics are contraindicated.

SPECIFIC ELECTROLYTE PROBLEMS

Sodium

Sodium is the major extracellular cation. Its movement is inextricably linked to that of water. Disorders of sodium balance are therefore the same as over- and under-hydration, and are dealt with earlier in this appendix.

Potassium

Unlike sodium, potassium is mainly an intracellular ion, and the small quantities measurable in the serum and extracellular fluid represent only a fraction of the total body potassium. However, the exact value of the serum potassium is important as cardiac arrhythmias can occur at values outside the normal range. As the majority of potassium is stored intracellularly, this acts as a large buffer to maintain the serum value within its normal narrow range. Thus, hypokalaemia is usually only manifest after significant total body depletion has occurred. Similarly, hyperkalaemia represents significant total body overload, beyond the ability of the kidney to compensate. The exception to both these statements is the situation in which the cell wall pumping mechanism is breached. A breakdown of the causes of hyper- and hypokalaemia is given in Table B.8.

Table B.8.   Causes of hypo- and hyperkalaemia

Hypokalaemia	Hyperkalaemia
Diarrhoea	Renal failure
Alkalosis	Acidosis
Volume depletion	Adrenal insufficiency
Primary hyperaldosteronism	Cell lysis
Diuretic abuse	Excessive potassium intake

Hypokalaemia

Hypokalaemia is rarely a great emergency. It is usually the result of excessive potassium losses from acute diarrhoeal illnesses. As total body depletion will have occurred, large amounts are required to return the serum potassium to normal. The fastest way of giving this is with oral supplementation. In cases where this is unlikely to be tolerated, intravenous supplements are required. However, strong potassium solutions are dangerous and can precipitate arrhythmias; thus the concentration of potassium in intravenous solutions ought not to exceed 80 mmol/l. Fortunately, this is not usually a problem as renal conservation of potassium aids restoration of normal serum levels.

Patients who are alkalotic, hyperglycaemic (but not diabetic), or are receiving insulin from exogenous sources, will have high intracellular potassium stores. Thus hypokalaemia in these cases is the result of a redistribution of potassium rather than potassium deficiency, and treatment of the underlying causes is indicated.

Hyperaldosteronism is a cause of hypokalaemic alkalosis. Patients with this condition will have salt and water retention, and will be hypertensive on presentation. Isolated hyperaldosteronism is the body's natural response to hypovolaemia and salt deficiency. Thus secondary hyperaldosteronism is a common cause of hypokalaemic alkalosis. As there is primary salt and water deficiency the patient is not usually hypertensive. The most common causes are diarrhoeal illness and salt-losing conditions such as cystic fibrosis. External loss of cerebrospinal fluid and fluid loss from intestinal ostomies or drains are other causes. Although potassium replacement is required in this condition, the main thrust of therapy has to be with salt and water replacement to re-expand the circulation and cut down on aldosterone production.

Hyperkalaemia

Hyperkalaemia is a dangerous condition. Although the normal range extends up to 5·5 mmol/l it is rare for arrhythmias to occur at levels below 7·5 mmol/l. The most common cause of hyperkalaemia is renal failure – either acute or chronic. Hyperkalaemia can also result from potassium overload, loss of potassium from cells due to acidosis or cell lysis, hypoaldosteronism, and hypoadrenalism.

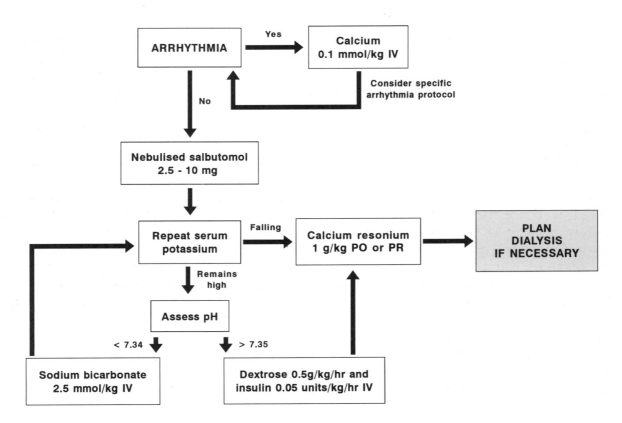

Figure B.2. Algorithm for the management of hyperkalaemia

The immediate treatment of hyperkalaemia is shown schematically in Figure B.2. If there is no immediate threat to the patient's life because of an arrhythmia, then a logical sequence of investigation and treatment can be followed. β_2-Stimulants, such as salbutamol, are the immediate treatment of choice for hyperkalaemia. They act by stimulating the cell wall pumping mechanism and promoting cellular potassium uptake. They are best administered by nebuliser. The dose to be given is shown in Table B.9. The serum potassium will fall by about 1 mmol/l with these dosages.

Table B.9. Salbutamol dose by age

Age (years)	Salbutamol dose (mg)
≤2·5	2·5
2·5–7·5	5
>7·5	10

Sodium bicarbonate is also effective at rapidly promoting intracellular potassium uptake. The effect is much greater in the acidotic patient (in whom the hyperkalaemia is likely to be secondary to movement of potassium out of the cells). The dosage is the same as that used for treating acidosis and 2·5 ml/kg of 8·4% $NaHCO_3$ is usually effective. It is mandatory also to check the serum calcium, because, particularly in patients with profound sepsis or renal failure, hyperkalaemia can be accompanied by marked hypocalcaemia. The use of bicarbonate in these situations can provoke a crisis by lowering the ionised calcium fraction, precipitating tetany, convulsions or hypotension, and arrhythmias.

Insulin and dextrose are the classic treatment for hyperkalaemia. They are not, however, without risks. It is very easy to precipitate hypoglycaemia if monitoring is not adequate. Large volumes of fluid are often used as a medium for the dextrose and, particularly in the patient with renal failure, hypervolaemia and dilutional hyponatraemia can then be a problem. Many patients are quite capable of significantly increasing endogenous insulin production in response to a glucose load, and this endogenous insulin is just as capable of promoting intracellular potassium uptake. It thus makes sense to start treatment with just an intravenous glucose load and then to add insulin as the blood sugar rises. The initial dosage of glucose ought to be 0·5 g/kg/hour, i.e. 2·5 ml/ kg/hour of 20% dextrose. Once the blood sugar is above 10 mmol/l, insulin can be added if the potassium is not falling. The dosage of insulin is initially half that used in diabetic ketoacidosis, i.e. 0·05 unit/kg/hour. This can then be titrated according to the blood sugar.

The above treatments are the fastest means of securing a fall in the serum potassium, but all work through a redistribution of the potassium into cells. Thus, the problem is merely delayed rather than treated in the patient with potassium overload. The only ways of removing potassium from the body are with dialysis or ion-exchange resins such as polystyrene sulphonate resins, e.g. Calcium Resonium. If it is anticipated that the problem of hyperkalaemia is going to persist, then the use of these treatments ought not to be delayed. Dialysis can only be started when in an appropriate environment. Ion-exchange resins can be used at the outset. The dosage of Calcium Resonium is 1 g/kg as an initial dose either orally or rectally, followed by 1 g/kg/day in divided doses.

In an emergency situation where there is an arrhythmia (heart block or ventricular arrhythmia), then the treatment of choice is intravenous calcium. This will stabilise the myocardium, but will have no effect on the serum potassium. Thus the treatments discussed above will still be necessary. The dosage is 0·5 ml/kg of 10% calcium gluconate (i.e. 0·1 mmol/kg Ca^{2+}). This dose can be repeated twice.

Calcium

Some mention of disorders of calcium metabolism is relevant as both hyper- and hypocalcaemia can produce profound clinical pictures.

Hypocalcaemia

Hypocalcaemia can be a part of any severe illness. Specific conditions that may give rise to hypocalcaemia include severe rickets, hypoparathyroidism, pancreatitis, rhabdomyolysis, and citrate infusion (in massive blood transfusions). Acute and chronic renal failure can also present with severe hypocalcaemia. In all cases hypocalcaemia can produce weakness, tetany, convulsions, hypotension, and arrhythmias. Treatment is that of the underlying condition. In the emergency situation, however, intravenous calcium can be administered. As most of the above conditions are associated with a total body depletion of calcium, and as the total body pool is so large, acute doses will often only have a transient effect on the serum calcium. Continuous infusions will often be required, and must be given through a central venous line because calcium is so irritant in peripheral veins. In renal failure, high serum phosphate levels may prevent the serum calcium from rising and dialysis is often indicated in these circumstances.

Hypercalcaemia

Hypercalcaemia usually presents as long-standing anorexia, malaise, weight loss, failure to thrive, and vomiting. Causes include hyperparathyroidism, hypervitaminosis D or A, idiopathic hypercalcaemia of infancy, malignancy, thiazide diuretic abuse, and skeletal disorders. Initial treatment is with volume expansion with normal (physiological) saline. Following this, investigation and specific treatment are indicated.

C

Child abuse

INTRODUCTION

All those working with children have an overwhelming impulse to deny that human beings will harm their young. Health care workers will come into contact with:

1. Children who have been abused by adults or by other children.
2. Children who have abused other children.
3. Adults who were abused as children.

In any group of staff up to 1% may have been abused themselves. If these survivors have had support following the abuse, they will be able to recognise and help abused children. If they have residual problems arising out of their own abuse, they may become disturbed and need help themselves if approached by children or adults whose experiences reflect their own.

Historical

The standard of care of children has varied over the centuries. Up to the nineteenth century, children were used in industry in a manner that today we would classify as abuse. In Victorian times beating children as a means of discipline was accepted by most social groups. Today, corporal punishment is forbidden in schools but the laws of the UK allow parents to administer physical punishment to children within limits.

A good working definition is that a child is considered to be abused if he or she is treated by an adult or by another child in a way that is unacceptable in a given culture at a given time.

The extremes of physical abuse were described in 1962 by Kempe, an American paediatrician, as the battered baby syndrome – multiple bruises, intracranial haemorrhages, fractures, and internal injuries in children under the age of 1 year. In Liverpool, between 1978 and 1987, there were five deaths of children under the age of 5 years due to similar injuries.

Since 1962 we have gradually recognised many more forms of abuse. Present classifications are as follows.

Classification of child abuse

Neglect

Neglect means the persistent or severe neglect of a child, or the failure to protect a child from exposure to any kind of danger, including cold or starvation, or extreme failure to carry out important aspects of care, resulting in the significant impairment of the child's health or development, including non-organic failure to thrive. There are at least 20 areas of care in which children may be neglected.

Physical injury

This is actual or probable physical injury to a child, or failure to prevent physical injury (or suffering) to a child, including deliberate poisoning, suffocation, and Munchhausen's syndrome by proxy.

Sexual abuse

This is the involvement of dependent, developmentally immature children, and adolescents in sexual activities which they do not truly comprehend, to which they are unable to give informed consent or which violate the social taboos of family roles. There are many types of sexual abuse:

- Touching, fondling, or licking of genitals or breasts.
- Masturbation of child by adult or adult by child; or of an adult in the presence of the child.
- Body contact with the adult genitals including rubbing or simulated intercourse by the adult against or between thighs, buttocks, or elsewhere.
- Heterosexual or homosexual intercourse with actual or attempted vaginal, anal, or oral penetration.
- Exhibitionism (the display of genitals).
- Involvement in pornography, including photography and erotic talk.
- Involvement in prostitution, male or female.
- Other varieties of sexual exploitation.

Most of these abusive acts will leave no physical signs on the victim.

Emotional abuse

This is described actual or probable severe adverse effect on the emotional and behavioural development of a child caused by persistent or severe emotional ill treatment or rejection. All abuse involves some emotional ill treatment. This category should be used where it is the main or sole form of abuse.

Grave concern

This is described in children whose situations do not currently fit the above categories, but where social and medical assessments indicate that they are at significant risk of abuse. These could include situations where another child in the household has been harmed or the household contains a known abuser.

Organised abuse

This characteristically involves multiple perpetrators, involves multiple victims, and is a form of organised crime. There are three sub-sections. The first is paedophile and/or pornographic rings. The second is cult-based ritualistic abuse in which the abuse has spiritual or social objectives. The third is pseudoritualistic abuse in which the degradation of children is the end rather than the means.

Presentations of physical abuse

- Head injuries – fractures, intracranial injury.
- Fractures of long bones
    - single fracture with multiple bruises;
    - multiple fractures in different stages of healing, possibly with no bruises or soft tissue injury;
    - metaphyseal or epiphyseal injuries, often multiple.
- Fractured ribs.
- Spinal injuries.
- Internal damage.
- Burns and scalds.
- Cold injury – hypothermia, frostbite.
- Poisoning – drugs or household substances.
- Suffocation.
- Cuts and bruises – imprints of hands, sticks, whips, belts, bites, etc. may be present.

Presentations of sexual abuse

- Disclosure by child.
- Suspicion by third party because of behaviour of child, especially changes in behaviour. These include: insecurity; fear of men; sleep disorders; mood changes, tantrums, aggression at home; anxiety, despair, withdrawal, secretiveness; poor peer relationships; lying, stealing, arson; school failure; eating disorders: anorexia, compulsive overeating; running away, truancy; suicide attempts, self-poisoning, self-mutilation, abuse of drugs, solvents, alcohol; unexplained acquisition of money; sexualised behaviour: drawings with a sexual content; knowledge of adult sexual behaviour shown in speech, play, or drawing; apparently sexual approaches; promiscuity.
- Symptoms such as sore bottom, vaginal discharge, bleeding per rectum, inflamed penis which caregiver believes is due to sexual abuse.
- Symptoms as above and/or signs, e.g. unexplained perineal tear and/or bruising, torn hymen, perineal warts, but doctor is the first person to suspect abuse.
- Sexually transmitted disease.
- Faecal soiling or relapse of enuresis.
- Child (usually adolescent girl) presents frequently with a variety of problems including: recurrent abdominal pain, overdose of drugs, reluctance to go home.
- Pregnancy but girl refuses to name the putative father or even indicate the category, e.g. boyfriend, casual acquaintance.

ASSESSMENT

The child who has disclosed abuse, or who is the subject of suspected abuse, will be overwhelmed by the number of professional people who are involved in the assessment of the situation. If the disclosure or suspicion arises in a nursery or school, then teachers and health visitors/school nurses will make preliminary enquiries and referrals. In all intra-familial abuse, social workers will speak to the child and the family. They will be responsible for the safety of the child, for ongoing care of the family, and for any subsequent civil proceedings. All child abuse is criminal activity so police officers will interview the alleged victim, the alleged offender, and any other witnesses to the incidents. In most areas of the UK good liaison exists between social workers and police officers so joint interviews are done to minimise the number of times the child will have to relate the details of the incident(s). Whenever possible, these interviews are recorded on video-tape to be used as evidence. Under the Criminal Justice Act 1991, video-tapes can be used as evidence in chief for children under the age of 14 years, provided that the child is available for cross-examination.

Medical assessment will be carried out by a paediatrician with forensic training or jointly by a police surgeon and a paediatrician. If the child has severe psychological disturbance or psychiatric symptoms, then a psychologist and/or psychiatrist will also see the child and the family. The basic medical assessment should follow the pattern used for all other diagnostic problems.

Details of medical assessment

History

Full details of the history of the incident(s) should be obtained from the child and the caregivers. If social workers and police officers have previously talked to the child, then taking this history from them may be appropriate, especially for alleged sexual offences. Frequent repetition of the details can be very disturbing to the child.

Systemic enquiry is then done for the cardiovascular system, respiratory system, gastrointestinal tract (remember to ask about soiling), urogenital system (remember to ask about wetting), central nervous system, musculoskeletal system, skin, and behaviour.

Personal history must start with pregnancy, birth, the neonatal period, and subsequent developmental milestones. Then details of immunisations, drug history, and allergies are obtained. Information on the child's performance at nursery or school should include social factors.

Enquiries are made about previous illnesses and injuries with dates of attendance at hospital or at the surgery of the family doctor. Whenever possible, past records should be obtained and relevant information should be extracted.

The traditional family history should include details of the natural parents, all cohabitees and any other people who regularly care for the child, e.g. relatives, childminders. Parental illness should be discussed, particularly psychiatric illness. Then the names, ages, and medical histories of all siblings and half-siblings are obtained. Any miscarriages, stillbirths, or deaths of siblings are discussed sensitively. Familial illnesses which are particularly important are inherited skin or blood disorders.

Examination

The general examination starts while the history is being taken. During that time the doctor observes the affect of the child, the relationships between child/mother/father/others present and any behavioural problems. If the child is reluctant to be examined, then playing with toys or the doctor's stethoscope often breaks the ice. No child should be examined against his or her will as this constitutes an assault. Sometimes a child who refuses to be examined one day will come back quite cheerfully another day. Examination under anaesthesia is rarely required.

Each child is examined from head to toe rather than in systems. Height and weight are checked, as is head circumference in babies. Careful notes are made of all normal and abnormal findings, including any marks on clothing, e.g. tears, blood stains. All marks, contusions, abrasions, and lacerations must be measured. Drawings must be made. If an abnormality is found that has not been discussed previously in the history, then further questions are asked – most undisclosed events are recent minor childhood accidents or previous ones that have left scars. When the upper part of the body has been examined, the child is asked to put the clothes back on to that area before taking the clothes off the abdomen and legs. Finally, the genitalia and anal region are examined. This method minimises the embarrassment of the sensitive child.

236

Investigations

During the examination, specimens needed for forensic investigation will be taken by a police surgeon or a paediatrician with forensic experience. These are relevant when there has been contact within 7 days of the examination. Swabs for microbiological investigation will be taken if there is a vaginal discharge or if threadworms may be present. Investigations for sexually transmitted diseases are done 2 weeks after the last alleged offence if oral, vaginal, or anal intercourse has taken place.

If bruises are found, then organic disease may be present with or without abuse, so haematological investigations are needed. Venous blood is taken for full blood count, bleeding, and clotting studies.

Plain radiographs are taken when a fracture or dislocation is suspected. In young children (usually under the age of 2 years) in whom physical abuse is suspected, a skeletal survey is done to diagnose multiple recent fractures and healed fractures. Sometimes an area of periosteal reaction is seen but no visible fracture line. This indicates that injury has occurred 10–14 days previously.

Diagnosis

Classic pointers to the diagnosis of inflicted injury are:

- There is delay in seeking medical help or medical help is not sought at all.
- The story of the "accident" is vague, is lacking in detail, and may vary with each telling and from person to person. Innocent accidents tend to have vivid accounts that ring true.
- The account of the accident is not compatible with the injury observed.
- The parents' affect is abnormal. Normal parents are full of anxiety for the child who has been injured. Abusing parents tend to be more preoccupied with their own problems – for example, how they can return home as soon as possible.
- The parents' behaviour gives cause for concern. They may become hostile, rebut accusations that have not been made, or leave before the consultant arrives.
- The child's appearance and his interaction with his parents are abnormal. He may look sad, withdrawn, or frightened. There may be visible evidence of a failure to thrive. Full-blown frozen watchfulness is a late stage and results from repetitive physical and emotional abuse over a period of time.
- The child may disclose abuse. Always make a point of talking to the child in a safe place in private if the child is old enough to be separated from the parents. Interviewing the child as an outpatient may fail to let the child open up as he is expecting to be returned home in the near future. He may disclose more in the safety of a foster home.

At the end of the medical assessment the diagnosis may be clear. More often the doctor has a differential diagnosis which includes abuse. Discussion then takes place between the social workers, health care workers, and police officers who have information about the family to balance the probabilities of abuse having occurred. In familial abuse a child protection conference will be held as soon as possible. In the meantime it may be necessary to arrange for the child to be taken to a place of safety (see "Emergency Protection Orders").

MANAGEMENT

All child protection work is based on cooperation between families, social workers, police officers, health care workers, and educationalists. This multi-agency approach is to ensure that all aspects of the care of the family are considered when decisions are being made. Certain decisions in management must be made by one profession, e.g. only a doctor can decide on the treatment required for fracture, only a police officer can decide the charge that is appropriate for the alleged offence. However, whenever possible, unilateral decisions are avoided in the best interests of the child and the family.

Some doctors are reluctant to share information with other professionals because of the ethical consideration of confidentiality. However, the Annual Standards Committee of the Council of the General Medical Council in November 1987 expressed the view that, if a doctor has reason for believing that a child is being physically or sexually abused, not only is it permissible for the doctor to disclose information to a third party but it is a duty of the doctor to do so. This is still the stance of the General Medical Council.

When the diagnosis is one of child abuse then the decisions to be made on management are the following:

- Does the child need admission for treatment of the injuries?
- Will the child be safe if returned home?
- If the child needs protection from an abuser who is in his or her own home, how can this be done?
- What support/protection is needed for the rest of the family?

If the alleged abuser is not in the same household as the child and the caregivers can protect the child, then he or she can return home. If the alleged abuser is in the same household as the child but is in custody, then the child will still be safe at home with another caregiver. When a person is charged and is allowed bail, one condition must be that he or she lives away from the household of the child. If this is not done then alternative care will be needed for the child.

Whenever there is a disclosure or suspicion of abuse, then the whole family needs support. Siblings may have been at risk of injury and so will need to be assessed. Spouses may be ambiguous in their loyalties to the child and to the alleged abuser. The child will need much support to withstand the stress of the investigation, especially if there are subsequent legal proceedings.

The details of management of these many facets are decided in the child protection conference. In this all the professional people meet with the family to collate information and to produce a plan of care.

MEDICOLEGAL ASPECTS

Health care professionals must be familiar with the medicolegal aspects of their work. The most important are the following:

- Emergency Protection Orders, Child Assessment Orders, Residence Orders, Police Protection Orders.
- Consent to examination.
- Writing of statements and reports for criminal and civil proceedings.
- Presentation of evidence.

Emergency Protection Order (EPO)

The Emergency Protection Order (Children Act 1989, sections 44 and 45) replaced the Place of Safety Order. It may be made for a maximum of 8 days with a possible further extension of up to 7 days. An application for discharge of that order may be made. Any person may apply for this order, but it will usually be an employee of the

NSPCC. The court may only make the order if it is satisfied that there is reasonable cause to believe that the child is likely to suffer significant harm if either he is not removed to another place or if his removal from a safe place (such as a hospital) is not prevented. Another clause is that, in the case of an application made by a Social Services Department or the NSPCC, the applicant "has reasonable cause to suspect that a child is suffering or is likely to suffer significant harm" and enquiries which are being made with respect to the child "are frustrated by access to the child being unreasonably refused" and the applicant believes that access is required as a matter of urgency.

Child Assessment Order (CAO)

This Order (Children Act 1989, section 43) addresses those situations where there is good cause to suspect that a child is suffering or is likely to suffer significant harm but is not at immediate risk, and the applicant believes that an assessment (medical, psychiatric, or other) is required. If the parents are unwilling to cooperate, the Social Services Department or the NSPCC can apply for a Child Assessment Order. The Order has a maximum duration of 7 days from the date on which it comes into effect. The court will direct the type and nature of the assessment that is to be carried out, and whether the child should be kept away from home for the purposes of the assessment. A child of reasonable understanding may refuse to have this assessment. Lawyers suggest that a child of reasonable understanding is a normal child of 10 years of age or more.

Residence Order

A Residence Order states with whom the child is to live. It has the effect of ending any care order and gives parental responsibility to the person with the order.

Police Protection Order

A constable has powers (Children Act 1989, section 46) to take a child "into police protection" for up to 72 hours. This power can be used to prevent the removal of a child from hospital.

Consent to examination

Consent for all examinations that are for evidential purposes must be obtained from a person with parental responsibility. In the Children Act 1989 (section 3), parental responsibility is defined as "all the rights, duties, powers, responsibilities and authority which by law a parent has in relation to the child and his property". Those with parental responsibility are specified in the Children Act 1989 (section 2). This can be summarised as in the box.

Parental responsibility

- Parents married at time of birth both have parental responsibility which continues after separation or divorce
- An unmarried mother has parental responsibility
- An unmarried father can apply to obtain parental responsibility; he can be appointed a guardian or if he can prove paternity then he can have the same legal position as if married
- Person in whose favour a Residence Order has been made – this is for the duration of the Order
- Appointed guardian
- Local Authority while a Care Order is in force
- Person who applies for an Emergency Protection Order

When more than one person has parental responsibility, each of them can act alone and without the other in meeting that responsibility. Parents do not lose parental responsibility if a Care Order or an Emergency Protection Order is in force. Parents lose parental responsibility with an Adoption Order. Parental responsibility can be delegated to a person acting on their behalf, e.g. while they are on holiday.

To cover emergency situations, those caring for a child who do not have parental responsibility may do what is reasonable in all the circumstances for the purpose of safeguarding or promoting the child's welfare.

Consent from the child or young person is needed if that person is of sufficient understanding to make an informed decision. Lawyers suggest that in a normal child this would be at age 10 years. The Gillick ruling (1986) allows an individual under the age of 16 years to submit to examination and treatment without the parents being informed, provided that is the wish of the child or young person.

Court reports

When preparing a written report on a child for the court all health care professionals should keep in mind that the written report may be used in subsequent court appearances. Therefore, the report should be confined to the facts. Whenever possible, objective and measurable evidence of the child's health and development should be presented. Where subjective views must be given they should reflect balanced professional judgement. If the report is comprehensive and comprehensible, then the health care professional may not be called to give verbal evidence in person. Always keep a copy of the report and a photocopy of the original notes if they have to be filed in a general filing system. All court personnel will ask for the original notes to be produced, but if these have gone missing then a photocopy may be acceptable. For the health care professional this is essential for good evidence.

Statements

The purpose of a statement is to provide the court with an informative and relevant account of the medical assessment of the child. The statement will give details of the persons involved, the observations, and the findings. Information given by another person should not be included unless this has been requested. In many areas, the Crown Prosecution Service wish statements to record all information although hearsay may be excluded before presentation to the court.

A statement is a professional document. It should be well written in good basic English. Technical terms should be avoided or, if quoted, should be followed immediately by appropriate lay terms. Most statements will be for the prosecution and a printed statement form will be provided. The standard sequence of writing a statement is as shown in the box.

Sequence for writing statement

1. Full name with surname in capitals
2. Qualifications
3. Occupation
4. Name of person requesting the assessment
5. Date, time, and place of the assessment
6. Name of person who was examined
7. Name of persons present
8. Details of the relevant history – if general history taken produced nothing significant then make a general comment including the sight of the detailed notes
9. Details of examination – if joint examination then specify who did each part
10. Investigations
11. Opinion on findings
12. The time at which examination ended

240

Each page must be signed at the bottom and the final page must be signed on the line below the completion of the writing. Any alterations must be initialled.

Always keep a copy of the statement.

Presentation of evidence

Dress in a professional manner. Arrive early in court. Take along all notes relevant to the case. Revise these on the day before the court proceedings. With permission from the magistrate or judge, you may refer to contemporaneous notes. However, revision helps to put the whole picture of the incident into the forefront of your mind so that you can find the appropriate notes more quickly.

When giving evidence stay calm even if the barrister becomes abusive. Do not be persuaded to answer questions which are outwith your knowledge or experience.

D

Childhood accidents and their prevention

INTRODUCTION

Child accident and injury prevention is important because of the following:

- On average, three children die in accidents every day.
- Accidents are the most common cause of death among children aged 1 to 14 years.
- Accidents cause half of all deaths of children aged between 10 and 14 years.
- Accidents result in about 10 000 children being permanently disabled annually.
- Accidents cause one child in five to attend an accident and emergency department every year.
- Accidents lead to one-fifth of all hospital paediatric admissions.

To put it another way, accidental injury to children leads to about 900 deaths, 120 000 hospital admissions and about 2 million accident and emergency department attendances in England and Wales every year.

This is the bad news about children's accidents. The good news is that they may often be prevented. This is because accidents are not unpredictable acts of God. They are closely linked to the child, his or her circumstances, and development. There are measures available that can prevent accidents completely or diminish their impact – measures that are applicable to a variety of fields.

RISK FACTORS

Who is most at risk? There are definite predisposing factors which enable high-risk groups to be identified.

Sex

Boys are more frequently injured than girls. The difference emerges at age 1–2 years. How much of this difference is innate and how much cultural is a subject for speculation. Girls may mature more rapidly in terms of perception and coordination.

Age

Children's accidents are intimately related to development. Take falls as an example. A newborn baby can only fall if dropped, or if a parent falls holding the baby. An older baby can wriggle and roll off a changing table or a bed. A crawling baby can climb upstairs and fall back. A small child can climb and fall out of a window. An older child can climb a tree, or fall in a playground. Knowledge of development helps in anticipation of dangers.

Exposure to different circumstances also varies with age. Children under 5 years experience accidents at home. School-age children experience accidents at school, sport, and play, and are especially at risk of accidental deaths as pedestrians.

Social class

As with so many other health problems, accidents are linked to inequalities in environments. Children in social class V, derived from head of household's occupation, are twice as likely to die from an accident as children in social class I and, for some accident types, such as burns, the chances are six times higher.

This does not mean that working-class parents care less about their children than middle-class parents, or that they do not know about accident risks. It may mean that there are many other pressures – overcrowding, lack of money, poor housing – and there is less power – owning one's own home, being able to afford safety equipment – to make changes for safety.

Psychological factors

Accidents are more common in families where there is stress from mental illness, marital discord, moving home, and a variety of similar factors.

Ethnic origin

On the whole, social class is more important than ethnic origin in determining accident risk.

ACCIDENT PREVENTION

How can injuries be prevented? There are a number of basic principles.

Accidents can be prevented completely. This is termed "primary prevention". An example is a fireguard preventing access to an open fire. The harm caused by an accident can be minimised. This is secondary prevention. For example, a seat belt can reduce injury even if a car crash occurs. Finally, rapid attention to an injury can reduce mortality and morbidity. This is tertiary prevention. Examples are cold water on burns and scalds, or pressing on a laceration.

There are three main approaches to accident prevention. These are the following.

Education

Increasing knowledge about a problem and the solutions, to change attitudes and eventually behaviour.

Engineering

Safe design of products and the environment, including the architecture of the home.

Enforcement

The role of legislation, regulations, and standards in accident prevention.
Countermeasures can be active, i.e. a conscious decision to use them has to be taken every time. This could be putting pans on the back hobs of the cooker. They can be passive, i.e. built in to the product. For example, junior formulations of paracetamol are sold in small bottles that do not contain a lethal dose.

How can doctors participate in reducing children's injuries? There are a variety of things they can do.

Be informed

This can be at a personal level. Most doctors could learn more about child safety from a Mothercare catalogue than they did as part of undergraduate or postgraduate education. Suggestions for reading are included in the box.

Set a good example

Wear your seat belt. Drive carefully past schools. Consider your own home and family with safety in mind.

Take opportunities

Can you offer safety advice to a family – or a whole ward – after an accident has happened? Do you know possible preventive strategies for that accident type? Have you developed the communication skills to listen to parents, and advise them?
Can you photograph that injured child in that setting, and use it to support a family in improving their household, or a neighbourhood in a media campaign?

Collaborate with others

Be prepared to participate in working groups and campaigns. You have special expertise and influence to offer.
Children's accidents and injuries are *the* major public health problem to children in Britain today. All doctors should learn more about them and have something to offer in reducing their toll.

SUGGESTED READING

Basic Principles of Child Accident Prevention – A Guide to Action. Child Accident Prevention Trust. London, 1989. (Available by post from CAPT, 28 Portland Place, London W1N 4DE. £6.00 inclusive of p.&p.)
Play it Safe. Dr Sara Levene. BBC Books. London, 1992. (A simple guide for all parents. Available from bookshops)

E

If you don't succeed

Each year, children are brought dead or dying into accident and emergency departments. Causes of sudden death in infancy include sudden infant death syndrome (SIDS) and congenital malformations, overwhelming infections, and child abuse. In older children, trauma, substance abuse, and pre-existing conditions such as myocarditis and idiopathic pulmonary hypertension may cause sudden death. Whatever the cause, the sudden death of a child is a disaster of overwhelming proportions for the parents at the time and in the long term.

When a doctor is told that an ambulance has brought a dead child to the hospital door, there is no place for certifying the child in the ambulance and then directing the ambulance to the mortuary. All such babies and children should be brought into the hospital, usually into the resuscitation room in the accident and emergency department to initiate the assessment and care of the child, and the support of the parents.

The initial assessment should be performed immediately by the accident and emergency doctor, while the parents are shown into a quiet room where a senior nurse should stay with them so that they do not feel isolated. If only one parent arrives, the other parent, or in the case of a single-parent family another appropriate person such as a relative or friend, should be contacted and asked to come to the hospital immediately.

The initial assessment establishes the need for resuscitation. If the child is being resuscitated by ambulance personnel as he or she arrives, this should be continued until a physical examination has taken place, and the decision to continue or not is formally made by the senior doctor leading the resuscitation. If the child is dead, as many victims of sudden infant death syndrome are on arrival at hospital, the physical examination and ECG, with full documentation, should still be performed. This should contain details of the state of dress, cleanliness, nutrition, presence of vomit or bleeding, or any signs of illness or injury. Local practice will dictate which swabs and specimens need to be taken and from which sites. In unexpected death the results of these may help elucidate the cause of death, e.g. infection or genetic disorder. Any attempts at resuscitation must also be documented. All this information will be needed by the pathologist and coroner who must later try to determine the cause of death and interpret any abnormal findings *post mortem*. Very occasionally a mother will refuse to let go of an obviously dead child, and the examination may have to be delayed for a short while or performed on the mother's knee.

Once the child has been declared dead, and in the absence of any suspicious circumstances, the nurses wash the child and dress him or her in clean clothes to make the child presentable for the parents to see. A shroud should not be used as this makes the body seem "untouchable" to many parents. Any discoloration of the skin or injuries can often be covered by a blanket. All the clothes and belongings brought with the child should be carefully placed in a bag and retained for the pathologist's examination. A photograph of the child should be taken in case the family do not have a picture of their child. Keep this photograph in the notes to be available in the future if it is needed.

As soon as the child is declared dead, the doctor must turn to the needs of the parents. The most senior doctor in charge of resuscitation who has had experience of deaths in children should undertake this task, together with the nurse who has been keeping vigil with the parents. In some hospitals an accident and emergency doctor is the appropriate person and in other hospitals a paediatrician undertakes this role.

The first task the doctor must perform, after introducing him- or herself to the parents, is to break the bad news, simply and sensitively but honestly and unambiguously. The parents usually know that the child is dead, but still have a glimmer of hope and wish for a miracle, especially after a blue-light ride in an ambulance and the admission of their child to a room full of high-tech equipment. They need to know that their child has "died" or "is dead", not "lost" or "slipped away". Some staff appear naturally to be better at breaking bad news than others, but techniques can be learned and experience gained. Simple measures help, such as being honest, sitting down at the same level as the parents, possibly touching, leaning forward and being attentive, not avoiding eye contact, but knowing when to look away.

The parents' reaction can vary from denial, anger, withdrawal, overt distress, to crying. It has been stated that no reaction is abnormal, each varying as the parent's personality, sex, culture, and previous life experience.

The doctor next needs to take as full a history as possible of the child and family. This helps the pathologist in assessing the possible cause of death. It also helps the parents to start exploring their own feelings of guilt, and allows the carer to begin the counselling.

The parents need to know about what will happen in the next few hours and days, and the doctor, nurse, or other appropriate person must start imparting this information. In some counties, the police accompany any 999 ambulance calls. This is routine, as is their practice of going into the home and obtaining details of the family and the circumstances of the child's death to aid the coroner's investigation. This in no way implies suspicion of the cause of death, but is routine, and the parents and relatives, and even the neighbours, need to know this. They also need to know that the coroner has to be informed routinely in this country of all cases of death by accident or injury, or where the cause of death is unknown or was sudden or unexplained. Again, this in no way implies suspicion of the parents. The coroner will ask for a postmortem examination to be performed by a pathologist of his or her choice, and may require the body to be transferred to an appropriate mortuary for this to take place. The parents need to know about the postmortem examination quickly as in some centres this takes place on the same day as the death. They have to be informed of the postmortem examination, not asked for their permission, and they often need a simple explanation of the procedure and the need for it. They should be told that it is necessary to try to find the cause of death, and that it is an examination similar to an operation performed by a doctor (a pathologist) in a careful respectful manner.

The parents need to be asked if they want a priest, vicar, or other religious leader to attend, and also to be asked about baptism. A service similar to baptism after death in the unbaptised child can give the parents great comfort. The parents should also know that the child can be dressed in his or her own clothes or accompanied by his or her favourite toy, even after death.

Most units have a social worker or member of staff who will give long-term support to the family. This person acts as a counsellor and friend of the family, and gradually takes over the care of both the child and the parents. She or he gives both emotional support and practical guidance for the first very traumatic hours and later for as long as the parents request it, sometimes for months or even years. She or he ensures that the parents have all the practical information they need at this trying time. This includes information booklets from the Department of Health on *What to do after a Death*, a Home Office guide on *The Work of the Coroner*, a booklet on grants for funeral costs, a parent information booklet on the Foundation for the Study of Infant Deaths and their 24-hour help-line telephone number, and the telephone numbers of the local bereavement groups. She or he also gives the hospital telephone number and her or his own name as a contact person. All information given is also written down, as the parents are often confused and bewildered, and cannot remember verbal instructions.

Before the parents leave the hospital, they should see and, if possible, feel able to touch and even cuddle their child. Very few do not wish to do this, and many studies have shown that, although at the time it appears to increase anguish and distress, parents benefit in the long term. It gives them a chance to face the reality of the child's death and to say goodbye. It also takes away the fantasy of how the body looks. Reality is much more manageable and acceptable than fantasy. Parents often like to see the child in the room where he or she died, especially if they were not present at the time of the death. It makes the parents feel closer to the event and even part of it. A nurse should sit with the child until the parents come, and she or he can do much to make the child's body more approachable to the parents, by touching the child as the parents enter. The parents may need to be told that it is alright to touch and hold their child as they feel powerless in the hospital situation. The nurse or doctor can help by saying something simple like "Would you like to see and cuddle _____ even if it is only to say goodbye". The parents may wish to spend some time alone with their child, but the attendant should not be too far away in case their distress becomes too great, or in case the mother suddenly wants to take her child away, as occasionally happens. Any other relatives present may also wish to see and hold the child.

Officially, the police need to identify formally any victims of sudden death. This may be done sensitively if the policeman or -woman is discretely present for a short time when the parents sit with the child.

The parents may find it difficult to leave the body or the place of death. They may wish to leave but may need a clear indication that it is alright to do so, or they may be naturally reluctant to leave their child and may need gentle persuasion after an appropriate time to do so. They need to know that they can return at any time before or after the postmortem examination to see their child, and that this is alright even if it is in the middle of the night. The parents should try to phone to give about an hour's notice, so that the body can be brought out of the mortuary and into the chapel of rest or other suitable place.

When the time comes for the parents to leave the hospital, they should have transport arranged for them. They should not drive in a state of shock, and they certainly should not have to travel on public transport if they have no transport of their own. They need a lift from a friend or relative, or a taxi, and, in the case of a single parent, they also need someone to accompany them and to stay with them.

The doctor has yet more duties to perform once the family has left the hospital. The whole case must be well documented, and this should include details of the parents and their reactions as well as the clinical details of the child. The doctor must then inform the Coroner or the Coroner's Office, the general practitioner and the Community Child Health Department, the health visitor, and the local hospital if the child is due to attend for an appointment. Ideally the general practitioner should visit the family soon after they return home to begin family support. If the mother was breastfeeding the child, she will also need treatment to suppress lactation.

If local arrangements allow, the parents should be told of the results of the postmortem examination as soon as possible after it has been completed, to relieve them of the suspense and some of the guilt.

In addition to all this initial management, there is much medium- and long-term work which would be of value to the family and could either be done by a nurse, social worker, or counsellor. Parents may need to know how to cope with the questions from relatives and friends, with the behaviour and questions of other children, and about the prospects of having other children and the outlook for them. Circumstances often change in families after a childhood death, and the family may need much counselling. Separation, divorce, a change of job, or a change of house is often observed in these families under stress. Ideally longer-term bereavement counselling should be arranged if and when the families will accept it. These families will need extra support and care particularly after the birth of any subsequent children.

CHECKLIST

The baby

- Full and thorough examination
- Core temperature
- Swabs – throat, nose, rectal
- Specimens – blood, etc. as local pathologist requests
- Keep clothes in labelled hospital bag
- Wrap baby in clean warm baby clothes for parents to hold
- Take photographs of baby and keep in notes

The parents

- Explain that the child (use name) has died and that nothing they could have done would have prevented it
- Gently get as full a history as possible
- Ask if they would like a priest/religious leader present
- Ask if they want any close relative to be contacted
- Encourage the parents to see and hold the baby
- Let them know the postmortem examination needs to be carried out
- Let them know that police are always informed of sudden unexpected deaths, and will need to ask a few simple questions of the carers
- Ask what address the family will be going to on leaving hospital
- Arrange transport from hospital to home and if alone make sure they are accompanied and not left alone at home

Be gentle, unhurried, calm and careful.
Do not guess at the diagnosis.

Obtain details of:

- Baby's and parents' names
- Baby's date of birth
- Address at which death occurred
- Time of arrival in department
- Time last seen alive
- Usual address if different from above

Inform

- GP of death and address to which parents will be going from hospital
- Health visitor
- Social worker
- Any relative as requested by the family
- Coroner – who will need to know the full name and address, and date of birth of child, time of arrival, place of death, brief recent history, any suspicious circumstances

---

At the end of a shift spent coping with the sudden death of a child in the accident and emergency department, staff will be under great stress. They should be supported in this work by being taught about it beforehand and by staff counselling sessions afterwards. The work is time-consuming and can be distressing but is a very worthwhile part of the work of an accident and emergency department.

A checklist is useful as a reminder of necessary actions for when a child is brought into hospital having died of an unknown cause (e.g. ?sudden infant death syndrome). An outline checklist is shown in the box.

The coroner will inform the police and pathologist.

F

Formulary

The formulary is intended as a reference to be used in conjunction with this book. To this end the drugs mentioned elsewhere are set out alphabetically below, along with their routes of administration, dosage and some notes on their use.

GENERAL GUIDANCE ON THE USE OF THE FORMULARY

The total daily dose of drugs is given. To calculate the actual dose given at each administration, divide the total daily dose by the number of times per day that the drug is to be given.

When dosage is calculated on a basis of per kilogram and a maximum dose is not stated, then the dose given should not exceed that for a 40 kg child.

The exact dose calculated on a basis of per kilogram may be difficult to administer because of the make-up of the formulations available. If this is the case the dose may be rounded up or down to a more manageable figure.

Doses in the formulary are sometimes written as µg or ng. When prescribing such doses these terms should be written in full (micrograms or nanograms respectively) in order to avoid confusion.

More detailed information about individual drugs is available from the manufacturers, from hospital drug information centres, and from the pharmacy departments of children's hospitals.

Abbreviations

The following abbreviations are used:

IM	intramuscular
IV	intravenous
SC	subcutaneous
via ETT	via the endotracheal tube

The final responsibility for delivery of the correct dose remains that of the physician prescribing and administering the drug.

253

Drug	Route	Total daily dose (TDD) 1 month to 12 years	< 1 month	Times daily (divide TDD by this figure)	Notes
Acyclovir Injection 250 mg, 500 mg vials	IV infusion	30 mg/kg	30 mg/kg	3	Antiviral Normal or immunocompromised. Administer over 1 hour in 5% dextrose or 0·9% saline. Reduce dose in mild renal impairment
Adenosine Injection 3 mg/ml vials	IV	50 µg/kg to a maximum total dose of 500 µg/kg	50 µg/kg to a maximum total dose of 250 µg/kg	Single dose	Antiarrhythmic Increase to 100 µg/kg then 250 µg/kg
		Effect enhanced by dipyridamole, antagonised by theophylline			
Adrenaline Injection 1:10 000 Minijet	IV	0·1 ml/kg of 1:10 000 (10 µg/kg) to a maximum dose of 10 ml of 1:10 000	0·1 ml/kg of 1:10 000 (10 µg/kg)	First dose	α and β sympathomimetic *Ventricular fibrillation, asystole and electromechanical dissociation.* IV doses may be given by intraosseous route flushed with 0·9% saline
		1 ml/kg of 1:10 000 (100 µg/kg)	0·1–0·3 ml/kg of 1:10 000 (10–30 µg/kg)	Subsequent doses	
Injection 1:1000 ampoules	via ETT	0·1 ml/kg of 1:1000 (100 µg/kg)	0·1 ml/kg of 1:1000 (100 µg/kg)	First and subsequent doses	Given via endotracheal tube
	IV infusion	500 ng/kg/min (30 µg/kg/h)	Use only with advice	Continuous	*Inotropic support* Starting dose. May be increased up to 2 µg/kg/min. Causes marked peripheral vasoconstriction
	IV	0·01 ml/kg of 1:1000 (10 µg/kg)	0·01 ml/kg of 1:1000 (10 µg/kg)	Single dose	*Acute anaphylaxis* Dose may be doubled and repeated
	IV infusion	0·1–5 µg/kg/min	0·1–5 µg/kg/min	Continuous	Anaphylaxis if bolus dose not effective
Use injection solution in nebuliser	Nebuliser	5 ml of 1:1000	Use only with advice	Single dose	*Croup* Dilute with 0·9% saline if required, for nebulisation. Repeat every 2–4 hours. Monitor ECG
		Inactivated by sodium bicarbonate			

continued

Note: Dose given is total daily dose unless otherwise stated.
If a maximum dose is not stated the dose given should not exceed that for a 40 kg child.

Drug	Route	Total daily dose (TDD) 1 month to 12 years	< 1 month	Times daily (divide TDD by this figure)	Notes
Alprostadil (prostaglandin E$_2$)					Prostaglandin
Injection 0·5 mg/ml ampoules (0·5 mg diluted to 500 ml = 1 µg/ml)	IV infusion	50–100 ng/kg/min (3–6 µg/kg/h) **then**	50–100 ng/kg/min (3–6 µg/kg/h) **then**	Continuous	Starting dose
		5–20 ng/kg/min (0·3–1·2 µg/kg/h)	5–20 ng/kg/min (0·3–1·2 µg/kg/h)	Continuous	Maintenance dose — Infuse in 5% dextrose or 0·9% saline. Apnoea may occur
Aminophylline					Bronchodilator
Injection 25 mg/ml ampoules	IV	5 mg/kg to a maximum dose of 250 mg	Use only with advice	Single dose	Loading dose over 15–30 minutes. If plasma level obtained give 1 mg/kg for 2 mg/l desired increase in level
	IV infusion	1 mg/kg/h	Use only with advice	Continuous	Maintenance dose. Dilute to 1 mg/ml in 5% dextrose or 0·9% saline

Monitor plasma levels. Reduce dose in liver disease. Note potential for drug interactions. Plasma levels increased by cimetidine, ciprofloxacin, and erythromycin

Drug	Route	TDD 1 month to 12 years	< 1 month	Times daily	Notes
Amiodarone					Antiarrhythmic
Injection 50 mg/ml ampoules	IV	5 mg/kg	Use only with advice	Single dose	Loading dose over 20–120 minutes at a concentration of up to 2·4 mg/ml in 5% dextrose only
	IV infusion	625 µg/kg/h (10 µg/kg/min)	Use only with advice	Continuous	

Caution in moderate renal impairment, risk of thyroid dysfunction with accumulation of iodine. Enhances effect of warfarin, increases levels of digoxin (halve maintenance dose), phenytoin, cyclosporin. Increased risk of bradycardia, atrioventricular block and myocardial depression with β-blockers, Ca^{2+} channel blockers. Additive effects with other antiarrhythmics. Toxicity increased with loop diuretics, cimetidine. Plasma level monitoring required

continued

Note: Dose given is total daily dose unless otherwise stated.
If a maximum dose is not stated the dose given should not exceed that for a 40 kg child.

Drug	Route	Total daily dose (TDD) 1 month to 12 years	< 1 month	Times daily (divide TDD by this figure)	Notes
Amoxycillin	IV	50–100 mg/kg to a maximum dose of 4 g		4	Antibiotic (penicillin) Bolus IV injection or short infusion in 5% dextrose or 0·9% saline over 30 minutes
			Up to 7 days 30 mg/kg	2	
			Over 7 days 30 mg/kg	3	
Reduce in severe renal impairment. Do not mix with aminoglycosides, flush line or separate by 30 minutes					
Ampicillin	IV	50–100 mg/kg to a maximum dose of 4 g		4	Antibiotic (penicillin) Dilute dose to twice volume and bolus over 3–5 minutes
			Up to 7 days 50–75 mg/kg	2	
			Over 7 days 75–100 mg/kg	3	
	IV infusion	400 mg/kg		4	Severe infection Infuse over 30 minutes
			Up to 7 days 100–150 mg/kg	2	
			Over 7 days 150–200 mg/kg	3	
Reduce dose in severe renal impairment. Do not mix with aminoglycosides, flush line or separate by 30 minutes					
Atropine sulphate Injection 100 µg/ml Minijet	IV	20 µg/kg (minimum 100 µg)	Do not use in neonates	Single dose	Antimuscarinic *Asystole and bradycardia.* Administer over 1 minute. IV doses may be given by the intraosseous route; 40 µg/kg may be given via endotracheal tube
Benzylpenicillin Injection 600 mg vials	IV infusion	300 mg/kg to a maximum dose of 12 g		6	Antibiotic (penicillin) *Dose for severe infection*
600 mg =1 megaunit =1 000 000 units			**Up to 7 days** 30 mg/kg	2	Infuse over 30 minutes to reduce irritation and CNS toxicity. Do not mix with aminoglycosides, flush line, or separate by 30 minutes
			Over 7 days 45 mg/kg	3	
Reduce dose in severe renal impairment, risk of convulsions					

continued

Note: Dose given is total daily dose unless otherwise stated.
If a maximum dose is not stated the dose given should not exceed that for a 40 kg child.

Drug	Route	Total daily dose (TDD) 1 month to 12 years	< 1 month	Times daily (divide TDD by this figure)	Notes
Bretylium Injection 50 mg/ml ampoules	IV	**Up to 12 years** Do not use **Over 12 years** 5–10 mg/kg	Do not use in neonates	Single dose	Antiarrhythmic Give over 10 minutes in 5% dextrose or 0·9% saline. May be repeated after 20 minutes, maximum 30 mg/kg/day. Monitor BP, ECG
	IV infusion	**Up to 12 years** Do not use **Over 12 years** 400 µg/kg/h	Do not use in neonates	Continuous	Maintenance dose

Caution increased myocardial depression with any combination of two or more antiarrhythmics. Enhanced hypotensive effect with anaesthetics, several other drug interactions – seek advice. Do not use in children under 12 years of age

Drug	Route	Total daily dose (TDD) 1 month to 12 years	< 1 month	Times daily	Notes
Bupivacaine (plain)					Local anaesthetic
	Local infiltration	Up to 2 mg/kg (0·8 ml/kg) to a maximum of 150 mg (60 ml of 0·25%)	Up to 2 mg/kg (0·8 ml/kg)	Single dose not more than every 8 hours	

Avoid or reduce dose in liver disease

Drug	Route	Total daily dose (TDD) 1 month to 12 years	< 1 month	Times daily	Notes
Calcium gluconate Injection 10% (100 mg/ml or 0·225 mmol Ca^{2+}/ml) ampoules	IV	0·07 mmol/kg (0·3 ml/kg of 10% injection)	0·02–0·05 mmol/kg (0·1–0·2 ml/kg of 10% injection)	Single dose	Acute calcium supplementation Slow IV injection
	IV infusion	1 mmol/kg (0·2 ml/kg/h of 10% injection)	1 mmol/kg (0·2 ml/kg/h of 10% injection)	Continuous over 24 hours	Maintenance infusion Dilute to at least 0·045 mmol/ml (20 mg/ml) with 5% dextrose or 0·9% saline, maximum infusion rate 0·0225 mmol/ml (10 mg/minute) *Electromechanical dissociation due to electrolyte imbalance*
	IV	0·225 mmol/kg (1 ml/kg of 10% injection)	0·225 mmol/kg (1 ml/kg of 10% injection)	Single dose	Administer slowly and check for bradycardia Can cause asystole. IV doses may be given by intraosseous route

Precipitates with sodium bicarbonate. Large doses of Ca^{2+} may cause arrhythmias with cardiac glycosides. Increased risk of hypercalcaemia with thiazide diuretics

continued

Note: Dose given is total daily dose unless otherwise stated.
If a maximum dose is not stated the dose given should not exceed that for a 40 kg child.

Drug	Route	Total daily dose (TDD) 1 month to 12 years	<1 month	Times daily (divide TDD by this figure)	Notes
Calcium chloride Injection 10% (100 mg/ml, 6·8 mmol Ca^{2+} in 10 ml) Minijet	IV infusion	1 mmol/kg	Do not use in neonates	Continuous	Calcium supplement Maintenance dose *Electromechanical dissociation due to electrolyte imbalance*
	IV	0·07–0·2 mmol/kg (0·1–0·3 ml/kg of 10% injection)	Do not use in neonates	Single dose	Slow injection IV doses may be given by the intraosseous route
Precipitates with sodium bicarbonate. Large doses of Ca^{2+} may cause arrhythmias with cardiac glycosides. Increased risk of hypercalcaemia with thiazide diuretics					
Calcium Resonium powder 1 level 5 ml spoonful=5 g	Oral or rectal	0·5–1 g/kg to a maximum of 60 g		3–4	Ion exchange resin for potassium removal Administer orally with a drink but not fruit squash (high in potassium). Rectal enema prepared by stirring powder into methylcellulose solution
Special rectal suspension			0·5 g/kg	Single dose	
Monitor calcium and potassium levels. Avoid use with aluminium- and magnesium-containing drugs. Caution with digoxin — levels may be increased. Inadequate dilution may cause impaction of resin					
Captopril Tablets 2 mg, 12·5 mg, 25 mg special powders	Oral	250–500 µg	Do not use in neonates	Test dose	Angiotensin-converting enzyme inhibitor Gradually increase to maintenance dose. Monitor blood pressure, renal function and electrolytes
Segments 0·5 mg, 1 mg, 6·25 mg	Oral	3 mg/kg	Do not use in neonates	3	Maintenance dose
Avoid or reduce dose in mild renal impairment, risk of hyperkalaemia. Many interactions including enhanced hypotensive effect with anaesthetics, antihypertensives, anxiolytics, hypnotics, diuretics, baclofen. Hypotensive effect antagonised by corticosteroids. Increased risk of hyperkalaemia with potassium-sparing diuretics, cyclosporin, potassium. May increase levels of digoxin and lithium. Seek further advice					
Cefotaxime Injection 500 mg, 1 g, 2 g vials	IV	100 mg/kg to a maximum dose of 2 g **then**		Initial dose **then**	Antibiotic (cephalosporin) Severe infection Given by short infusion

continued

Note: Dose given is total daily dose unless otherwise stated.
If a maximum dose is not stated the dose given should not exceed that for a 40 kg child.

Drug	Route	Total daily dose (TDD) 1 month to 12 years	< 1 month	Times daily (divide TDD by this figure)	Notes
Cefotaxime (contd)		200 mg/kg to a maximum dose of 12 g		Subsequent doses 4	Give by short infusion
			Up to 7 days 100 mg/kg	2	Infection
			Over 7 days 150 mg/kg	3	
		Reduce dose in severe renal impairment. Bolus over 3–5 minutes or dilute 4–10 times with infusion fluid and administer over 20–60 minutes. Do not mix with aminoglycosides			
Ceftazidime Injection 500 mg, 1 g, 2 g vials Injection 250 mg vials	IV	150 mg/kg to a maximum dose of 9 g	60–100 mg/kg	3 2	Antibiotic (cephalsporin) Severe infection Infection
		Reduce dose in mild renal impairment. Administer over 5–10 minutes as IV bolus or 20 minutes as short infusion. Do not mix with aminoglycosides			
Cefuroxime Injection 250 mg, 750 mg, 1·5 g vials	IV (IM)	100 mg/kg to a maximum dose of 4·5 g		3–4	Antibiotic (cephalosporin) Bolus over 3–5 minutes
			100 mg/kg	3	
					Severe infection
	IV infusion	200 mg/kg to a maximum dose of 9 g		3	Infuse over 20–30 minutes in 5% dextrose or 0·9% saline
		Reduce dose in mild renal impairment. Do not mix with aminoglycosides			
Chloramphenicol Injection 1 g vials	IV	25 mg/kg **then** 75 mg/kg		Initial dose 4	Antibiotic (aminoglycoside) *Severe infection*
	IV		12·5 mg/kg	Single dose	Monitor levels and seek advice on size and frequency of dose
		IM absorption variable. Avoid in severe renal impairment and liver disease. Monitor levels and full blood count. Increases levels of many drugs including phenytoin and warfarin. Chloramphenicol levels decreased by phenobarbitone			

continued

Note: Dose given is total daily dose unless otherwise stated.

If a maximum dose is not stated the dose given should not exceed that for a 40 kg child.

Drug	Route	Total daily dose (TDD) 1 month to 12 years	< 1 month	Times daily (divide TDD by this figure)	Notes
Chlorpheniramine Injection 25 mg/ml	IV	**1 month–1 year** 250 µg/kg	Do not use in neonates	Single dose	Sedative antihistamine Repeat up to four times in 24 hours if necessary. Dilute with 5–10 ml water for injection or 0·9% saline and give over 1 minute. May cause transient drowsiness, giddiness and hypotension especially if administered too rapidly
		1–5 years 2·5–5 mg		Single dose	
		6–12 years 5–10 mg to a maximum of 20 mg		Single dose	
		Avoid in liver disease, may produce coma			
Clonazepam Injection 1 mg/ml ampoules	IV	50 µg/kg to a maximum of 1 mg	Use only with advice	Single dose	Benzodiazepine Administer slowly
	IV infusion	10 µg/kg/h	Use only with advice	Continuous	Dilute with 5% dextrose or 0·9% saline
		Reduce dose in severe renal impairment. May produce coma in liver disease. Respiratory depression possible with IV administration. Enhanced sedative effects with anaesthetics, opioid analgesics, antihistamines, antidepressants, α-blockers, antipsychotics, baclofen, nabilone, cimetidine			
Desferrioxamine Injection 500 mg vials	Oral	5–10 g	Use only with advice	Single dose (in 50–100 ml water)	Iron-chelating compound Leave dose in stomach after lavage. Injection solution may be given orally – unpleasant taste
	IM	1–2 g to a maximum dose of 2 g	Use only with advice	Single dose	To eliminate iron already absorbed. If shocked, hypotensive or seriously ill administer IV. Dose may be repeated every 3–12 hours to a maximum of 6 g/day for adults
	IV infusion	Up to 15 mg/kg/h (maximum 80 mg/kg/day)	Use only with advice	Continuous	Decrease rate after 4–6 hours to ensure daily maximum not exceeded. Continue until serum iron less than total iron-binding capacity. Reconstitute 500 mg with 5 ml water for injection and infuse in 5% dextrose or 0·9% saline
		Incompatible with heparin. Caution: anaphylaxis and hypotension from rapid IV injection. Use with caution in renal impairment			

continued

Note: Dose given is total daily dose unless otherwise stated.
If a maximum dose is not stated the dose given should not exceed that for a 40 kg child.

Drug	Route	Total daily dose (TDD) 1 month to 12 years	< 1 month	Times daily (divide TDD by this figure)	Notes
Dexamethasone					
Injection dexamethasone phosphate 8 mg in 2 ml (equivalent to 6·7 mg base in 2 ml); 4 mg in 1 ml (equivalent to 3·3 mg base in 1 ml)	IV	600 µg/kg	600 µg/kg	4	Corticosteroid – glucocorticoid Meningitis to reduce meningeal inflammation and incidence of severe hearing loss. Usually given for 4 days. Bolus over 3–5 minutes. Infusion in 5% dextrose or 0·9% saline
All doses are quoted as base	Reduces effects of rifampicin and antiepileptics; antagonises effects of diuretics and antidiabetics. High doses may cause Cushing's syndrome. Withdraw gradually to avoid acute adrenal insufficiency. May suppress growth and increase risk of infection				
Diazepam					
Diazepam injection 5 mg/ml ampoules	IV	250–400 µg/kg	200 µg/kg	Single dose	Benzodiazepine Slow IV bolus over 3–5 minutes. Repeat after 10 minutes if necessary
Diazepam in lipid emulsion for injection 5 mg/ml ampoules		**then** 100–400 µg/kg/h	**then** 5–20 µg/kg/h	**then** continuous	Use diazepam in 5% dextrose or 0·9% saline for central lines, maximum concentration 80 mg/l. Use diazepam in lipid emulsion in 5% dextrose or 0·9% saline for bolus, in 5% dextrose only for continuous infusion at maximum concentration 400 mg/l, into peripheral lines. In severe fluid restriction 1 mg/ml has been used
Rectal solution 5 mg/2·5 ml, 10 mg/2·5 ml	Rectal	**Up to 1 year** 2·5 mg **1–3 years** 5 mg **4–12 years** 5–10 mg to a maximum dose of 10 mg	2·5 mg	Single dose Single dose Single dose	Repeat dose if necessary after 5 minutes
	Caution: in liver disease, may precipitate coma. Reduce dose in severe renal impairment. Beware respiratory depression in acute use – antagonist flumazenil. Enhanced sedative effects with anaesthetics, opioid analgesics, isoniazid, antihistamines, α-blockers, antihypertensives, baclofen, ulcer healing drugs, omeprazole. Seek advice				

continued

Note: Dose given is total daily dose unless otherwise stated.
If a maximum dose is not stated the dose given should not exceed that for a 40 kg child.

Drug	Route	Total daily dose (TDD) 1 month to 12 years	< 1 month	Times daily (divide TDD by this figure)	Notes
Digoxin Tablets 62·5 µg, 125 µg, 250 µg Elixir (liquid) 50 µg/ml	Oral, IV (IM)	30 µg/kg	30 µg/kg	3 for 24 hours	Cardiac glycoside Digitalisation (loading dose). Slow IV over 5 minutes or short infusion over 30 minutes in 5% dextrose or 0·9% saline. Vasoconstriction from rapid injection. Decrease loading dose if cardiac glycosides received in last 2 weeks
Injection 100 µg/ml, 250 µg/ml ampoules	Oral (IM)	8 µg/kg (maximum 250 µg/dose)	8 µg/kg (maximum 250 µg/dose)	2	Maintenance Monitor plasma levels and adjust dose as necessary
		Reduce dose in mild renal impairment. Increased levels with amiodarone, diltiazem, verapamil, quinidine, quinine, and low serum potassium. Increased prolonged levels with erythromycin and tetracycline. Seek advice. Changing from IV to oral; increase dose of oral liquid by 20% and tablets by 30% to achieve same levels			
Dobutamine Injection 250 mg in 20 ml vials	IV infusion	2–10 µg/kg/min (120–600 µg/kg/h)	2–10 µg/kg/min (120–600 µg/kg/h)	Continuous	Inotrope Can be increased up to 40 µg/kg/min. Infuse in 5% dextrose or 0·9% saline
		Inactivated by sodium bicarbonate. Caution several drug interactions including hypertensive crisis with monoamine oxidase inhibitors. Seek further advice			
Dopamine	IV	1–5 µg/kg/min	1–5 µg/kg/min	Continuous	Inotrope *Renal dose – renal vasodilatation*
Injection 40 mg/ml ampoules	IV infusion	5–20 µg/kg/min	5–20 µg/kg/min	Continuous	Direct inotropic effect
		Infuse in 5% dextrose or 0·9% saline. Inactivated by sodium bicarbonate. Caution several drug interactions including hypertensive crisis with monoamine oxidase inhibitors. Seek further advice			
Enalapril					Angiotensin-converting enzyme inhibitor
Tablets 2·5 mg, 5 mg Special segments, powders	Oral	100 µg/kg to a maximum dose of 5 mg	Do not use in neonates	1	Starting dose
					Gradually increases until required effect achieved
		300 µg/kg to a maximum dose of 20 mg		1	Maintenance dose
		Avoid in neonates after arch surgery especially with large doses of diuretics. Avoid or reduce dose in mild renal impairment – risk of hyperkalaemia. Many drug interactions including enhanced hypotensive effect with anaesthetics, antihypertensives, anxiolytics, hypnotics, diuretics, baclofen. Hypotensive effect antagonised by corticosteroids. Risk of hyperkalaemia with potassium-sparing diuretics, cyclosporin, and potassium. Increase lithium concentrations. Seek further advice			

continued

Note: Dose given is total daily dose unless otherwise stated.
If a maximum dose is not stated the dose given should not exceed that for a 40 kg child.

Drug	Route	Total daily dose (TDD) 1 month to 12 years	< 1 month	Times daily (divide TDD by this figure)	Notes
Enoximone Injection 5 mg/ml ampoules	IV infusion	5–20 µg/kg/min (0·3–1·2 mg/kg/h)	Do not use in neonates	Continuous	Phosphodiesterase inhibitor Must be diluted with an equal volume of 0·9% saline or water for injection. Adjust dose according to response
Erythromycin Injection 1 g vials (lactobionate)	IV infusion	50–100 mg/kg to a maximum of 4 g	50 mg/kg	4	Antibiotic (macrolide) Dilute injection 10 times with 5% dextrose or 0·9% saline, infuse over 15–60 minutes
		Reduce dose in severe renal impairment, use with caution in liver disease. Drug interactions include increased levels of warfarin, carbamazepine, midazolam, digoxin, cyclosporin, theophyllines, disopyramide, alfentanil. Avoid use with terfenadine (metabolism inhibited, arrhythmias possible). Seek advice			
Flecainide Injection 10 mg/ml ampoules	IV	2 mg/kg to a maximum of 150 mg	Do not use in neonates	Single dose	Antiarrhythmic IV bolus over 20 minutes or dilute in 5% dextrose or 0·9% saline and infuse over 30 minutes at a concentration of 0·3 mg/ml. Monitor ECG
		Reduce dose in mild renal impairment. Avoid or reduce dose in liver disease. Drug interactions include increased levels with amiodarone and cimetidine, increased myocardial depression with any antiarrhythmic. Toxicity increased in hypokalaemia, e.g. with diuretics. Monitor plasma levels			
Flucloxacillin Injection 250 mg, 500 mg vials	IV	50–100 mg/kg to a maximum of 4 g		4	Antibiotic (penicillin) IV can be further diluted to twice the volume in 5% dextrose or 0·9% saline, bolus over 3–5 minutes
			Up to 7 days 50–75 mg/kg	2	
			Over 7 days 75–100 mg/kg	3	
		Do not mix with aminoglycosides, flush line or separate by 30 minutes			
Flumazenil Injection 100 µg/ml ampoules	IV	**Up to 1 year** 50 µg **1–7 years** 100 µg **7–12 years** 150 µg to a maximum dose of 200 µg	Do not use in neonates	Single dose	Benzodiazepine antagonist Initial dose over 15 seconds
		Up to 1 year 25 µg **1–7 years** 50 µg **7–12 years** 75 µg to a maximum dose of 100 µg	Do not use in neonates	Single dose	Repeat dose to be given at 1-minute intervals to maximum dose of 1 mg (2 mg in intensive therapy unit)
		Limited experience in children. Doses quoted for children are derived from adult dose and mean surface area. Contraindicated in prolonged benzodiazepine use in epilepsy			

continued

Note: Dose given is total daily dose unless otherwise stated.
If a maximum dose is not stated the dose given should not exceed that for a 40 kg child.

Drug	Route	Total daily dose (TDD) 1 month to 12 years	<1 month	Times daily (divide TDD by this figure)	Notes
Frusemide					Diuretic (loop)
Injection 10 mg/ml ampoules	IV	1 mg/kg to a maximum dose of 40 mg	1 mg/kg	Single dose	Maximum 4 mg/kg/dose
	IV infusion	0·1–4 mg/kg/h	0·1–4 mg/kg/h	Continuous	Infuse in 0·9% saline and not 5% dextrose
		Caution: in moderate renal impairment, may need higher doses. Deafness may follow rapid IV injection. May cause hypokalaemia — which may precipitate coma in liver disease. Drug interactions include increased risk of nephrotoxicity with non-steroidal anti-inflammatory drugs and ototoxicity with aminoglycosides, polymyxins, and vancomycin. Antagonises antidiabetic drugs, increases lithium toxicity. Toxicity of cardiovascular drugs and corticosteroids increased in hypokalaemia			
Gentamicin					Antibiotic (aminoglycoside)
Injection 10 mg/ml vials	IV (IM)	7·5 mg/kg		3	*Infection*
			Up to 7 days		
			<2 kg		IV bolus over 3–5 minutes or
			3 mg/kg	Single dose	short infusion over 20 minutes
			>2 kg		in 5% dextrose or 0·9% saline
			6 mg/kg	2	
			Over 7 days		
			<2 kg		
			6 mg/kg	2	
			>2 kg		
			7·5 mg/kg	3	
40 mg/ml vials	IV	9 mg/kg		3	*Cystic fibrosis or pyrexia in neutropenia*
		Do not mix with penicillins, cephalosporins, erythromycin. Flush between doses or separate by 30 minutes. Monitor plasma levels. Reduce dose in mild renal impairment. Increased risk of oto- and/or nephrotoxicity with cephalosporins, colistin, polymyxins, amphotericin, cyclosporin, vancomycin, loop diuretics, and in renal impairment. Enhances effects of tubocurarine. Contraindicated in myasthenia gravis			
Hydrocortisone					Corticosteroid
Injection 100 mg (as sodium succinate= Efcortelan, Solu-Cortef) (as sodium phosphate =Efcortesol)	IV (IM)	4 mg/kg	2·5 mg/kg	Single dose	Initial dose
		then	**then**	**then**	Maintenance dose. Repeat every 6 hours. Slow IV over 1–5 minutes. May be mixed with 5% dextrose or 0·9% saline. IV doses may be given by intraosseous route
		2–4 mg/kg	2 mg/kg	single dose	
Ipratropium bromide					Antimuscarinic bronchodilator
Atrovent 20 µg/ activation, Atrovent Forte 40 µg/activation	Nebuliser	**Up to 7 years** 125 µg	Do not use in neonates	3–4	Nebuliser solution may be diluted with 0·9% saline and/or mixed immediately before use with other nebuliser solutions except sodium cromoglycate
		Over 7 years 250 µg		3–4	

continued

Note: Dose given is total daily dose unless otherwise stated.
If a maximum dose is not stated the dose given should not exceed that for a 40 kg child.

Drug	Route	Total daily dose (TDD) 1 month to 12 years	< 1 month	Times daily (divide TDD by this figure)	Notes
Ipratropium bromide (contd) Nebuliser solution 250 µg/ml (100 µg in 0·4 ml) [prescribe in 25 µg (0·1 ml) multiples]	Oral inhalation (aerosol)	Up to 160 µg/day (8 puffs)	Do not use in neonates	3—4	Inhaler may be used with Nebuhaler (with mask for young children)
Dry mouth, urinary retention, constipation can occur					
Isoprenaline Injection 20 µg/ml Minijet	IV	5 µg/kg	5 µg/kg	Single dose	Sympathomimetic IV dose may be given by the intraosseous route
Injection 200 µg/ml or 1 mg/ml ampoules	IV infusion	1·2—12 µg/kg/h (20—200 ng/kg/min)	1·2—12 µg/kg/h (20—200 ng/kg/min)	Continuous	Starting dose, increase if necessary to 1000 ng (1 µg)/kg/min. Infuse in 5% dextrose or 0·9% saline at concentration of 4 µg/ml
Several drug interactions including increased risk of arrhythmias with volatile anaesthetics. Seek further advice					
Labetolol Injection 5 mg/ml ampoules	IV	250—500 µg/kg to a maximum dose of 50 mg	Do not use in neonates	Single dose	β-Blocker Loading dose
	IV infusion	30 µg/kg/min (1·8 mg/kg/h)	Do not use in neonates	Continuous	Starting maintenance dose. Infuse in 5% dextrose or 0·9% saline at a concentration of 1 mg/ml. Must have arterial pressure monitoring. May require atropine to counteract severe bradycardia
Avoid in liver disease, can cause severe hepatocellular injury. Several drug interactions including enhanced hypotensive effect with anaesthetics, other antihypertensives, anxiolytics, hypnotics, and diuretics. Hypotensive effect antagonised by non-steroidal anti-inflammatory drugs, corticosteroids, sympathomimetics. Increased risk of myocardial depression and bradycardia with antiarrhythmics. Risk of heart block with amiodarone, diltiazem. Severe hypotension and heart failure may occur with nifedipine, verapamil. Increased atrioventricular block and bradycardia with digoxin. Seek further advice					

continued

Note: Dose given is total daily dose unless otherwise stated.

If a maximum dose is not stated the dose given should not exceed that for a 40 kg child.

Drug	Route	Total daily dose (TDD) 1 month to 12 years	< 1 month	Times daily (divide TDD by this figure)	Notes
Lignocaine					*Ventricular fibrillation or tachycardia*
Injection 20 mg/ml (2%) Minijet	IV	1 mg/kg to a maximum dose of 100 mg	1 mg/kg	Single dose	If necessary repeat every 5 minutes to maximum 3 mg/kg. IV dose may be given by the intraosseous route; 2 mg/kg may be given via endotracheal tube
					Antiarrhythmic
Injection 5 mg/ml (0·5%), 10 mg/ml (1%), 20 mg/ml (2%) ampoules	IV	0·5–1 mg/kg to a maximum dose of 100 mg	0·5–1 mg/kg to a maximum dose of 100 mg	Single dose	Loading dose. Administer over 1 minute
	IV infusion	10–50 µg/kg/min	10–50 µg/kg/min	Continuous	Maintenance dose. Infuse in 5% dextrose or 0·9% saline at a concentration of 2 mg/ml
	Local infiltration	Up to 3 mg/kg	Up to 3 mg/kg	Single dose not more than every 4 hours	*Local anaesthetic*
Avoid or reduce dose in severe liver disease. Several drug interactions including increased myocardial depression with other anti-arrhythmics, β-blockers. Effect antagonised by hypokalaemia, e.g. with loop and thiazide diuretics. Metabolism inhibited by cimetidine. Seek further advice					
Mannitol Injection 10%, 20% infusion	IV infusion	0·5–1 g/kg	Do not use in neonates	Single dose over 1 hour	Diuretic (osmotic) May be repeated once or twice after 4–8 hours
Morphine					Opiate
Injection 2·5 mg/ml, 10 mg/ml ampoules	IV	**1–3 months** 25 µg/kg	25 µg/kg	Single dose	Repeat up to four times in 24 hours
		3–6 months 50 µg/kg		Single dose	Repeat up to four times in 24 hours
		Over 6 months 100 µg/kg		Single dose	Repeat up to six times in 24 hours
	IV infusion	**1–6 months** 5 µg/kg/h	5 µg/kg/h	Continuous	Administer IV bolus first as loading dose. Infuse in 5% dextrose or 0·9% saline
		Over 6 months 10 µg/kg/h		Continuous	
Causes constipation and nausea. Avoid in moderate renal impairment and in liver disease (can precipitate coma). Caution: enhances sedative effects of anxiolytics and hypnotics; antagonises effects of cisapride and metoclopramide. Morphine levels increased by cimetidine. Can cause respiratory depression. Antagonist is naloxone					

continued

Note: Dose given is total daily dose unless otherwise stated.
If a maximum dose is not stated the dose given should not exceed that for a 40 kg child.

Drug	Route	Total daily dose (TDD) 1 month to 12 years	< 1 month	Times daily (divide TDD by this figure)	Notes
Naloxone					Opiate antagonist
Injection 20 µg/ml, 400 µg/ml	IV	10 µg/kg	10 µg/kg	First dose	Give higher dose if response to first dose is inadequate
		then	**then**	**then**	
		< 20 kg 100 µg/kg	100 µg/kg	single dose	Repeat doses as necessary to maintain opioid reversal. May be given IM, SC or by intraosseous route if IV not possible
		> 20 kg 2 mg		single dose	
	IV infusion	5–20 µg/kg/h	5–20 µg/kg/h	Continuous	Half-life of opioid may be longer than that of naloxone. Consider infusion in 5% dextrose or 0·9% saline at concentration 4 µg/ml. Adjust rate as required
Nitroglycerin					Vasodilator
Glyceryl trinitrate injection 500 µg/ml 5 mg/ml ampoules	IV infusion	200–500 ng/kg/min (12–30 µg/kg/h)	Do not use in neonates	Continuous	Infuse in 5% dextrose or 0·9% saline. Administer via polyethylene tubing
Paracetamol					Analgesic and antipyretic
Suspension 120 mg/5 ml, 250 mg/5 ml Tablets 500 mg Dispersible tablets 500 mg Suppositories 125 mg, 250 mg, 500 mg	Oral or rectal	**1–2 months** Do not use **2–3 months** 10–15 mg/kg **Over 3 months** 15 mg/kg to a maximum dose 0·5–1 g	Do not use in neonates	Single dose Single dose	Repeat if necessary after 4–6 hours
		Avoid large doses in liver disease – dose-related toxicity			
Paraldehyde (injection used rectally)	Rectal	0·4 ml/kg to a maximum dose 5–10 ml	0·3 ml/kg	Single dose	Antiepileptic Dilute with an equal volume of arachis oil. May cause rectal irritation
Injection paraldehyde BP ampoules	IV infusion	1–4 ml/kg/h of a 5% solution		Continuous	Dilute 2·5 ml paraldehyde to 50 ml with 5% dextrose or 0·9% saline to produce 5% solution
		Use plastic syringe if administered within 10 minutes			

continued

Note: Dose given is total daily dose unless otherwise stated.
If a maximum dose is not stated the dose given should not exceed that for a 40 kg child.

267

Drug	Route	Total daily dose (TDD) 1 month to 12 years	< 1 month	Times daily (divide TDD by this figure)	Notes
Phenobarbitone Injection 30 mg/ml, 60 mg/ml ampoules	IV	15 mg/kg **then**	15–20 ml/kg	Single dose	Antiepileptic Administer over 5 minutes. Higher doses have been given to ventilated neonates
Mixture (alcohol free)	IV or oral	10 ml/kg to a maximum dose of 600 mg	8–10 ml/kg	2	Maintenance dose

Requires drug level monitoring. Avoid administration via umbilical artery cannulae in neonates due to alkalinity. Use with caution in liver disease – may precipitate coma. Reduce dose in severe renal impairment. Enzyme inducer with many drug interactions including a reduced effect of oral anticoagulants, griseofulvin, calcium channel blockers, corticosteroids, cyclosporin, theophylline, and thyroxine. Toxicity may be enhanced by other anticonvulsants without increase in efficacy. Antagonised by antipsychotics

Drug	Route	TDD 1 month to 12 years	< 1 month	Times daily	Notes
Phenytoin Phenytoin sodium injection 50 mg/ml ampoules	IV **then**	18 mg/kg **then**	18 mg/kg **then**	Single dose	Antiepileptic *Status epilepticus* (only to be given if not currently on phenytoin or if level less than 2·5 mg/l). Loading dose over 20–30 minutes
Phenytoin sodium 100 mg = 90 mg phenytoin base	IV infusion	8 mg/kg to a maximum of 400 mg	8 mg/kg	2	Maintenance dose. If plasma level 10–20 mg/l 2 hours after infusion, start maintenance dose 12 hours after loading dose complete. If less than 10 mg/l give further 5 mg/kg at once and start maintenance dose 8 hours after loading dose complete. IV infusion at not more than 1 mg/kg/min to avoid arrhythmias and hypotension. Cardiac monitoring essential. Maximum concentration 1 mg/ml in 0·9% saline only
	IV **then**	18 mg/kg **then**	18 mg/kg **then**	Single dose	*Antiarrhythmic* Loading dose
	IV infusion	5 mg/kg	5 mg/kg	Single dose	Maintenance dose. Infuse over 20–30 minutes in 0·9% saline only at maximum concentration 1 mg/ml with ECG monitoring. Monitor plasma levels

Reduce dose in liver disease. Concomitant administration of antiepileptic drugs may increase toxicity without increase in antiepileptic effect. Several drug interactions including increased levels with cimetidine, diltiazem. Enzyme inducer – reduces levels of phenobarbitone, carbamazepine, sodium valproate. Seek further advice

continued

Note: Dose given is total daily dose unless otherwise stated.
If a maximum dose is not stated the dose given should not exceed that for a 40 kg child.

Drug	Route	Total daily dose (TDD) 1 month to 12 years	< 1 month	Times daily (divide TDD by this figure)	Notes
Potassium chloride					Potassium supplement
Injection 2 mmol/ml (potassium chloride strong 15% w/v)	IV infusion	0·5 mmol/kg/h	0·5 mmol/kg/h	Single dose	Administer in 5% dextrose or 0·9% saline. Shake well to avoid layering. Up to 2 mmol/kg/h have been given in cardiac intensive care
	IV infusion	0·08 mmol/kg/h (2 mmol/kg in 24 h)	0·08 mmol/kg/h (2 mmol/kg in 24 h)	Continuous	Maintenance dose

Usual maximum concentration 4 mmol/100 ml and rate not more than 0·5 mmol/kg/h. Monitor electrolyte status and ECG. Avoid routine use in moderate renal impairment – high risk of hyperkalaemia. Increased risk of hyperkalaemia with angiotensin-converting enzyme inhibitors, cyclosporin, and potassium-sparing diuretics, e.g. amiloride. Caution: hyperkalaemia may lead to decreased digoxin levels

Drug	Route	Total daily dose (TDD) 1 month to 12 years	< 1 month	Times daily (divide TDD by this figure)	Notes
Prednisolone					Glucocorticosteroid
Tablets 1 mg, 5 mg, 25 mg		1–2 mg/kg	1–2 mg/kg	1–3	
Tablets (soluble) 5 mg, tablets (enteric-coated) 2·5 mg, 5 mg	Oral	2 mg/kg to a maximum dose of 60 mg	Do not use in neonates	1 or 2	Treat for 3–5 days then stop (no need to taper dose). To be taken in the morning or twice daily, with or after food

Reduces effects of rifampicin, antiepileptics. Effects of diuretics and antidiabetics antagonised

Drug	Route	Total daily dose (TDD) 1 month to 12 years	< 1 month	Times daily (divide TDD by this figure)	Notes
Propranolol Injection 1 mg/ml ampoules					β-Blocker *Cyanotic spells in Fallot's tetralogy*
	IV	100 µg/kg	30 µg/kg	Single dose	Inject slowly under ECG control. Indicated in, repeat as necessary up to 3 or 4 times daily May be used in dysrhythmias, phaeochromocytoma, thyrotoxicosis
	IV	10–50 µg/kg to a maximum dose of 1 mg	10–50 µg/kg	Single dose	*Dysrhythmias* Repeat as necessary up to 3 or 4 times daily

Administer IV slowly with ECG monitoring. Caution in severe renal impairment. May decrease renal blood flow. Reduce oral dose in liver disease. Avoid with verapamil. Seek advice on drug interactions

continued

Note: Dose given is total daily dose unless otherwise stated.
If a maximum dose is not stated the dose given should not exceed that for a 40 kg child.

Drug	Route	Total daily dose (TDD) 1 month to 12 years	< 1 month	Times daily (divide TDD by this figure)	Notes
Salbutamol					Selective β-adrenoceptor stimulant. Bronchodilator
Nebules 2·5 mg in 2·5 ml, 5 mg in 2·5 ml	Nebuliser	**Up to 6 months** Do not use	Do not use in neonates		Repeat up to 8 times per day, or 12 times per day in hospital with monitoring. Dilute to 3–4 ml with 0·9% saline. May be mixed with ipratropium, beclomethasone, budesonide, or sodium cromoglycate nebuliser solutions
		6 months–5 years 2·5 mg		Single dose	
		Over 5 years 5 mg to a maximum dose of 10 mg		Single dose	
Inhaler and Autohaler 100 µg per activation	Oral inhalation (aerosol or powder)	**Up to 6 months** Do not use	Do not use in neonates		Maximum acute treatment doses. Infants and children less than 2 years should use large volume spacer with mask, 2–5 years a large volume spacer is recommended, 5–12 years a spacer, dry powder or autohaler
Ventodisk 200 µg, 400 µg powder for use in Diskhaler		**6 months–2 years** Up to 2400 µg		6	
		3–4 years Up to 3600 µg		6	
		Over 5 years Up to 7200 µg		6	
Rotacaps 200 µg, 400 µg powder for use in Rotahaler	Oral inhalation (aerosol or powder)	**Up to 7 years** 200–400 µg	Do not use in neonates	Single dose	Emergency initial treatment doses A maximum of 400–600 µg can be given in 4 hours
		Over 7 years 200–600 µg		Single dose	A maximum of 800–1200 µg can be given in 4 hours
					100 µg via a large volume spacer can be administered every few seconds until improvement occurs. Use a mask for very young children
Injection 500 µg/ml ampoules	IV	5 µg/kg	Use only with advice	Single dose	Status asthmaticus or hyperkalaemia Bolus injection over 5–10 minutes. Repeat if necessary

continued

Note: Dose given is total daily dose unless otherwise stated.
If a maximum dose is not stated the dose given should not exceed that for a 40 kg child.

Drug	Route	Total daily dose (TDD) 1 month to 12 years	< 1 month	Times daily (divide TDD by this figure)	Notes
Salbutamol (contd)					
Injection for infusion 1 mg/ml ampoules	IV infusion	6–24 µg/kg/h (100–400 ng/kg/min)	Use only with advice	Continuous	Infusion in 5% dextrose or 0·9% saline at a concentration of 10 µg/mL. Doses have been doubled
		Caution: potentially serious hypokalaemia especially in severe asthma. Potentiated by theophylline, diuretics, corticosteroids, hypoxia. Monitor plasma potassium in severe asthma. Efficacy under 18 months of age uncertain			
Sodium bicarbonate					Alkylating agent
Injection 8·4% Minijet	IV	2·5 mmol/kg (2·5 ml/kg of 8·4%)	2·5 mmol/kg (2·5 ml/kg of 8·4%)	Single dose	*Acidosis and hyperkalaemia*
1 mmol/ml		1 mmol/kg (1 ml/kg of 8·4%)	1 mmol/kg (1 ml/kg of 8·4%)	Single dose	*Asystole*
					Dilute to 4·2% in 0·9% saline or water for injections
		Repeat as required. Administer slowly. Monitor blood gases, pH. Inactivates sympathomimetics such as adrenaline, dopamine			
Sodium nitroprusside					Vasodilator
Injection 50 mg ampoules	IV	500 ng/kg/min (30 µg/kg/h)	Use only with advice	Continuous	Starting dose
	IV infusion	200 ng/kg/min to a maximum dose of 6 µg/kg/min	Use only with advice	Continuous	Incremental dose
		Infuse in 5% dextrose or 0·9% saline at a concentration of 0·2–0·8 mg/ml; rate to be determined by continuous BP monitoring. Avoid prolonged use in moderate renal failure, avoid in liver disease. Enhanced hypotensive effect with anaesthetics, non-steroidal anti-inflammatory drugs, antihypertensives, anxiolytics, hypnotics, diuretics, baclofen. Antagonised by corticosteroids			
Verapamil					Calcium channel blocker
Injection 2·5 mg/ml ampoules	IV infusion	**Up to 1 year** Do not use	Do not use in neonates		Antiarrhythmic
		Over 1 year 15–100 µg/kg to a maximum dose of 10 mg		Single dose	Administer over 10 minutes. Monitor ECG
		Many drug interactions including increased hypotensive effect of general anaesthetics and risk of atrioventricular delay, increased risk of amiodarone-induced bradycardia, atrioventricular block, and myocardial depression. Increases levels of quinidine (extreme hypotension), tricyclics. Enhances effect of digoxin (atrioventricular block and bradycardia), carbamazepine, cyclosporin, lithium, non-depolarising muscle relaxants, theophylline. Decreased levels with rifampicin, reduced effect with phenytoin. Enhanced hypotensive effect with antipsychotics, severe hypotension, and heart failure with β-blockers. Seek further advice			

Note: Dose given is total daily dose unless otherwise stated.
If a maximum dose is not stated the dose given should not exceed that for a 40 kg child.

INDEX